THE HD DIET

THE HD DIET

Achieve Lifelong Weight Loss with Chia Seeds and Nature's Water-Absorbent Foods

KEREN GILBERT, MS, RD

RODALE.

Rodale books may be purchased for business or promotional use or for special sales.
For information, please write to:
Special Markets Department, Rodale Inc., 733 Third Avenue, New York, NY 10017

Printed in the United States of America
Rodale Inc. makes every effort to use acid-free ♾, recycled paper ♻.

Book design by Christina Gaugler

Library of Congress Cataloging-in-Publication Data is on file with the publisher.
ISBN 978-1-62336-293-5 hardcover

Distributed to the trade by Macmillan
2 4 6 8 10 9 7 5 3 1 hardcover

RODALE.

We inspire and enable people to improve their lives and the world around them.
rodalebooks.com

To my boys: Jonathan, Jake, Derek, and Kane

CONTENTS

ACKNOWLEDGMENTS ix

INTRODUCTION xi

P1 YOUR DECISION

Chapter 1: Hydrate and Satiate: The HD Philosophy 3

Chapter 2: Deciding to Live in HD 21

Chapter 3: Daily HD Decisions—Uncovering Your Current Habits 27

Chapter 4: Put It in Writing—Your HD Work 43

P2 THE 12-WEEK HD PLAN

Chapter 5: Eating in HD—The HD Plan Guidelines and Core Foods 65

Chapter 6: Start Strong in HD—Daily Checklists and Menus 89

Chapter 7: Still Focused and Adding IFs 109

P3 LIVING IN HD

Chapter 8: Healthy HD Alterations 131

Chapter 9: Curing Excusitis 145

Chapter 10: Meal Prep in HD 157

Chapter 11: The HD Recipes 171

AFTERWORD 237

APPENDIX A: MY HD CONTRACT 238

APPENDIX B: HD FOOD LOG 240

APPENDIX C: WEEKLY GOAL TRACKER 242

APPENDIX D: NAVIGATING THE SUPERMARKET 243

ENDNOTES 251

INDEX 252

ACKNOWLEDGMENTS

There are many people to acknowledge for their unwavering encouragement and advice in making *The HD Diet* a reality.

First, I would like to express my sincere gratitude to my agent Melissa Flashman. Your enthusiasm and vision for *The HD Diet* means the world to me. I felt a connection with you the moment I met you.

To Valerie Peterson: You just "got me" from the start and for that I will be forever appreciative.

To my team at Rodale: It has truly been an honor to work with you. To my editor Ursula Cary, your continued support, expertise, and guidance have been cherished throughout this journey. Thank you also to Jess Fromm, Marilyn Hauptly, Susan Turner, and Anastasiya Ganeeva for all of your assistance.

To Megan Hustad: Thank goodness for your exceptional organizational skills, continuous support, and, of course, your calming voice.

To Brad Behar: It's so nice to have a lawyer you trust and adore. Thank you for all of the hard work you have done for Decision Nutrition and *The HD Diet.*

To Dave Concannon: The best fitness trainer around and the one who helped me name my practice Decision Nutrition during one of our sessions. Thanks for the direction.

To Randy: Thank you for your vision and all the hours in the kitchen supporting Decision Nutrition.

To Harvey and Debra: I am so thankful for your food manufacturing expertise, honesty, and hard work.

To Susan and Jon: I am so appreciative for your enthusiasm and loyalty.

To Pam and Justin Fries: I thank you for conceptualizing with me the vision I had for my practice on a park bench. You never know when there will be a turning point in your life and you were there.

To Jennifer Goldberg: I have always been in awe of your entrepreneurial spirit. I thank you for always believing in me.

Barbra Berwald Dietz: I value you and your advice. You are infectious to be around. Your work ethic is inspiring. I thank you for all your support in this process and always.

To the best in-laws a girl can have: Jerry, you have always had faith in me and knew I can make a success of Decision Nutrition. Your support has been invaluable, not to mention you are the finest chia bagel delivery boy in the tri-state area. Gilda, you are an exceptionally modern woman who by her actions has shown me how to be a strong, tenacious woman.

To Sharone: Thank you for always being so creative and an abstract thinker, which has made me think out of the box many times.

To my mom: You have always been there to encourage me to reach for the stars and always love me unconditionally. You have taught me the true definition of selfless love. To my dad: I am so thankful for your advice, guidance, and support on this journey. Your thirst for knowledge and passion for Decision Nutrition and the HD plan has been my saving grace. Your faith in me has been a precious gift I will cherish forever. I love you, mom and dad!

To all of my clients who have made the decision to walk through my office door: Thank you for inspiring me at work each and every day. You gave me the courage to write this book and taught me what it is to live my life in HD. I sincerely thank you from the bottom of my heart. A special thanks to all the clients that have contributed to *The HD Diet*. I know your stories will inspire others to live their life in HD.

Finally, I must acknowledge the boys in my life. To my amazing husband, Jonathan: Words can't express my love and gratitude for you. Like on one of our long jogs together, you always have my back, push me forward and I go to places I never imagined I was capable of. I am blessed I found my best friend and soul mate to live decisively with—forever. And to the three boys we created: Jake, Derek, and Kane, you give me inspiration to better myself each and every day and fill my life with love and laughter. You can do anything in this life—you just need to decide!

INTRODUCTION

You wouldn't dream of buying a new television that wasn't in HD, right? It's only natural to want everything clear and sharply detailed. I believe we should all be living our lives in high definition, experiencing every moment in focus. But sometimes we can feel like fuzzy little dots meshed together, a grainy picture that only reflects a semblance of who we are. While everybody's issues are different, many of us feel that extra pounds are what "fuzz" us up. When we're not at our best weight, our best selves seem somehow obscured. We dress to hide, not to impress; we shrink into the background rather than shine the way we should. And even our best moments aren't as clearly enjoyable as they could be if we were more comfortable with ourselves.

If you've made the decision to open this book, it's likely because you're looking to lose weight. Perhaps you have been labeled "the fat one" in the family and have long struggled with extra pounds. Maybe you're in one of those tough transitional phases, like postbaby or pre-menopause. Or you could be experiencing the temptations of college dorm life. Maybe the stress of your family responsibilities is weighing you down—literally. Or maybe you've always been athletic and now you don't know why the beer belly isn't coming off.

As a nutritionist with a specialty in weight loss, I've learned from years of working with clients that everyone's struggles are different. As a working mother of three, I can tell you what my own are, and each person who comes into the Decision Nutrition office experiences her own personal journey. Like fingerprints and snowflakes, no two are exactly alike. But what my successful clients all have in common is this: Once they've made the first important *decision*—to walk through the door to my practice, to learn how to live in HD—they keep making the decisions that will lead them to their weight-loss goals. Making any sort of change entails *living decisively* in each moment. It means definitively saying "Yes!" to what works and "No, thanks" to what will likely derail you from your chosen path.

Some prospective clients have been to other nutritionists before me, constantly searching for the latest thing that will help them lose weight. These "fad-diet junkies" come to the first consultation based on a recommendation from a successful client or because they've heard about my reputation, and they think I'll have the proverbial magic pill. And, in truth, anyone can take my HD plan and a bag of chia seeds and run with it for a couple of weeks to drop some quick pounds. But I break the news to them that there is no magic wand you can just wave over yourself—or pay someone to wave at you—for lasting weight loss. I tell them, as I tell all my clients, that living life in HD means making the decision to be engaged with the process because it takes commitment and, even with the most effective diet, the journey isn't linear. There will always be bumps in the road.

Before I started Decision Nutrition, I had my own indecisive journeys and false starts. I stumbled through various identities: reluctant premed student; dedicated-but-unfulfilled institutional nutritionist; young, overwhelmed stay-at-home wife and mother; even a stint as an actress. I've felt the despair of losing myself, of trying hard to be what I thought others wanted me to be, knowing those roles weren't quite right, that I could be something more. I didn't quite have the courage or the knowledge or the skills to make a change, to do what I needed to do, to plant the stake of my best self into the ground.

I want to share with you a turning point in my life—an aha moment, as Oprah used to say. I was pregnant for the third time with my son Kane. My other sons, Jake and Derek, were 6 and 9 already, and getting pregnant again was not in my plan. I had loved being a young mom, but my boys were both in school now and getting more self-sufficient, and I had just begun to explore my own identity again. I took acting lessons (something I had always dreamed of) in addition to counseling people toward their health goals at two local gyms, in Starbucks, in my home, or anywhere a client wanted to meet. I was hungry to build myself up after feeling like the years had escaped me. I had lost focus. I felt fuzzy, and I wanted to feel clear. I wanted to live life in HD.

So, alas, the news of being pregnant again sent me spiraling into a negative place. How was I going to continue my journey to find myself with a young infant to take care of yet again? I was on the couch with my husband, Jonathan, pregnant and feeling sorry for myself, when I had my aha moment. I flipped my inner light switch and decided this baby was going to be my motivation. I had continually felt that my dreams and passions were being disrupted by events in my life. Well, getting pregnant for the third time didn't derail me; it propelled me to make the decision to start the business I had always dreamed of.

I was ready to create a nutrition consulting practice where I could help people be their best high-definition selves. Once I got clarity and committed to starting Decision Nutrition, so much of what I wanted fell into place.

It didn't happen overnight though. I began practicing in a little office within an office that I subleased from a chiropractor in Great Neck, Long Island. The main area was occupied by his billing department personnel and, for reasons unknown to me, two very unfriendly women. It was a good location and all I could afford, but these two officemates of mine created quite a hostile work environment for me. With subtle gestures and sneers, they made it clear that they were not thrilled about sharing their previously private lair with me. They would ignore me and would even shut off the lights when they left for the day (always before I was ready to leave) so that when I left my office in the evening, I would be enveloped in pitch-black. I learned to look past all of this and focus on myself and my practice. I marketed myself by running ads, partnering with local doctors and gyms, offering coupon specials, you name it! I worked on my Web site and developed my own materials, and I waited. Slowly, I began to get clients. Many came in because of the promises of free consultations and discounted sessions. I didn't care. I was happy as long as I was working consistently. I knew that I could have a positive impact on people with my ideas, which had been dormant for so many years.

I was fully engaged in the process. I learned to implement my philosophies. I worked, explored, and solicited. There were bumps in the road, for sure, but I just kept making the decisions necessary to work through my doubts every day. My research led me to develop the HD plan. My community embraced me, my business, and my principals and encouraged me to develop my own line of foods (my Decision Nutrition Chia Bagels and Chia Chips are an HD plan favorite). And my clients' life-changing successes remind me each day that I'm doing what I was meant to do; in fact, my clients encouraged me to write this book. I still work in the same building, but after 2 years I moved into my own office with my own waiting room. I've been in this office for 3 years, and when I work late, I walk out into a bright, cheerful environment—no more darkness.

A major component of my 12-week HD plan is learning how to incorporate *hydrophilic,* or "water loving," foods (like oats, beans, and certain fruits and vegetables) and "hydro-boosting" chia seeds, which are high in water-soluble fiber, into your diet. *HD* stands for *hydrophilic diet*, but it also is the automatically recognizable acronym for *high definition.* Aha! The term *HD* was intriguing to me, and it illustrated the importance of how we should all feel. It also represented how I began to feel after starting Decision Nutrition. Thereafter, I would begin my client sessions with the statement, "You have to follow the HD to live in HD."

And my clients *do* change. During the 12 weeks of the HD plan, they reprogram their deeply ingrained lifestyles so that they think differently about what to eat and when to eat. They learn to regularly eat the right food combinations to stay satisfied while losing weight. And they learn to indulge in their IFs (infrequent foods) without guilt—"IF" they do it occasionally, with the intention to truly enjoy the indulgence. My clients have taken off baby weight; they have dropped weight during menopause; they have lost the "spare tire" that marathon training didn't get rid of. And they have kept the weight off. They've learned to feel better and to look better, and they've brought this success into other parts of their lives. They've learned to live life in high definition. You'll read about their experiences here, and you'll experience this, too, if you make the decision to lose weight and live in HD.

But to live your life 20 or 30 or 50 or more pounds thinner, you must first make the decision that this is what you want, that you deserve this. You have to decide that you will put the effort, the action, and the discipline into achieving it. And as you chart your way to a healthier, better-looking you, this book will be your road map. I will give you the tools and the encouragement you need to achieve your new high-definition reality. However, nobody but *you* can decide to make the journey. And once you do, you'll learn—as I did—that you can't go back to living in fuzziness.

In this book, you'll find the complete HD plan that I developed for my clients along with the coaching and stories that have helped my clients reach and maintain their goal weights. But opening a book, like stepping into a nutritionist's office, is the easy part. Are you ready to make the decision to uncover your best, healthiest self? Are you ready to *live decisively* in HD?

P1

YOUR DECISION

1

HYDRATE AND SATIATE— **THE HD PHILOSOPHY**

"Let your medicine be your food and your food be your medicine."
—HIPPOCRATES

Isn't it unbelievable that the Greek doctor Hippocrates wrote the quote above more than 2,000 years ago? I picture Hippocrates watching his overweight peers suffer from heart attacks and diabetes and hypothesizing that their ill health might not be caused by a curse from the gods but rather a lifestyle of meat, cheese, and wine orgies. Given all the knowledge we've gathered since then, it's amazing that we still struggle with the idea of food as healing. The Internet puts information about lifestyle and diet right at our fingertips, but so many of us resist the simple truth that our decisions about what to put in our bodies has a tremendous impact on our health, weight, and happiness.

Let's also not forget that we are constantly confronted by food decisions in our daily routines. Believe me, this occurs many more times than you might think! A study at Cornell University addressed exactly this issue. When 139 participants were asked how many food decisions they made in a typical day, the average answer given was 14. But when asked to consider daily choices as to when, what, how much, where, and who with to eat for every meal, snack, and drink, the number came out to a staggering 226 food decisions a day.[1]

As a nutritionist and registered dietitian, I take Hippocrates's words to heart. My vision has always been to help people improve their lives through the food decisions they make. Hey, we make so many food decisions that knowing what to eat can really be an overwhelming task for some people. It's my hope that by the end of this book, you won't feel overwhelmed, you'll understand how to incorporate hydrophilic foods into your diet, and you'll be living in HD.

Now what do I mean by hydrophilic foods? It was during my research to find the optimum healthy, beneficial foods to recommend to my clients (an ongoing quest!) that I first came across the word. *Hydrophilic* originates from the Greek words for water (*hydro*) and friendship (*philia*).

The word made me think of waves crashing on the shore and children frolicking in turquoise pools. It sounded fresh, clean, and hopeful. When applied to food, it is equally positive. A food is hydrophilic if it is "water loving," meaning it has a strong affinity for water. Hydrophilic foods fill up with water, and in turn, they fill you up, leaving you feeling satisfied.

I loved the idea, but I wanted a more in-depth understanding of how the science related to foods we ingest every day. I soon discovered that foods with a high hydrophilic quality contain an aquatic fiber known more commonly as soluble fiber. Now, we have been told over and over again to increase our fiber intake. *But all fiber is not created equal.* All fiber comes from the edible portion of plant cell walls. (I'm talking about foods like grains, nuts, seeds, fruits, and vegetables.) And all fiber is resistant to digestion to some degree. But there are *two* kinds of fiber: insoluble and soluble.

Understanding the distinction between water-insoluble and water-soluble (or hydrophilic) fiber is what led to my revolutionary HD plan.

ALMIGHTY FIBER

Hippocrates may have been one of the first on record to stress how food affects our health, but in the 1970s the surgeon Denis P. Burkitt pointed out some new angles. He compared the pattern of diseases in African hospitals with Western diseases and concluded that many diseases seen infrequently in Africa were the result of Western diets and lifestyles.[2] He noted that in cultures with diets rich in plant foods and fiber—like those in Africa—the medical conditions of diverticulitis, gallbladder disease, irritable bowel syndrome, heart disease, constipation, and colon polyps were rarely seen. His 1979 book, *Don't Forget Fibre in Your Diet,* became a bestseller.

Dr. Burkitt also illustrated that the diseases just mentioned largely emerged—and became big public health problems—in the United States and England after 1890. He concluded that this seemed to be associated with a new milling process that yielded a refined white flour—one that, you guessed it, is low in both soluble and insoluble fiber. A lot of research done in the past several decades confirms Dr. Burkitt's theory that consuming too much refined flour is detrimental to your health. (More to come on that when I talk about processed foods and how we need to stay away, in Chapter 7.)

Profound evidence that fiber is important for our health was also demonstrated in the work of the biochemist T. Colin Campbell in *The China Study*, coauthored with his son Thomas M. Campbell II. They found the average fiber intake in China to be about three times higher than in the United States. China also has lower incidences of colon and rectal cancers, and cholesterol levels are lower there as well. The lesson Dr. Campbell stresses is that the incredible abundance of processed and fast foods we enjoy in America has dire consequences for our overall well-being.

We have so many food decisions to make each day that it's hard to be consistently smart about what we eat, and it's easy to literally eat ourselves sick. The US health care system can attest to that. The medical care costs of obesity in the United States are astonishing. According to the Centers for Disease Control and Prevention, in 2008 these costs totaled about $147 *billion.*

So I am pretty certain that if one of the participants in Dr. Campbell's study hopped on a plane to the United States and started eating like we do, this person would likely put on an extra 20 pounds pretty quickly. The point is, we need to start eating more mindfully, with a focus on whole, healthful, hydrophilic foods that help us feel and look better inside and out.

How Much Fiber Do You Need?

How much fiber is ideal? The Institute of Medicine gives the following daily recommendations for adults.

	AGE 50 OR YOUNGER	AGE 51 OR OLDER
Men	38 grams	30 grams
Women	25 grams	21 grams

Most of us in the United States get 15 grams a day, according to the USDA. That's 10 grams less than the daily recommendation for women age 50 and under and more than 20 grams less for men in the same age range! I see this below-average intake of fiber with my clients when they first sit down with me to talk about their current dietary habits. They have been educated about fiber and know it can be associated with health benefits, including weight loss. But they still struggle to lose those stubborn pounds.

So what's the problem? First, there's some confusion about what foods contain fiber. I can't tell you how many times I have been asked how much fiber is in a serving of milk or a piece of fish. Here's the answer: No animal products contain fiber! Second, as mentioned earlier, there are two kinds of fiber—insoluble and soluble—and they each contribute to different health benefits. While people know about fiber generally, they don't know much about *what kind of fiber* to up their intake of. There are no USDA guidelines to tell you if your daily diet needs more insoluble fiber, soluble fiber, or both. I think this is the culprit of ongoing weight struggles for so many people.

To keep pounds away, you need to focus on the hydrophilic (water-loving) fiber. This will lead to what I call HD satiation, which leads to shedding those excess pounds. Satiety is the key to long-term weight management success.

Insoluble Fiber: Sweepers and Water-Phobes

These are fibers that do not dissolve in water. They pass through our digestive system close to their original form. The scientific names for insoluble fibers include cellulose and lignins, and most of them come from the bran layers of cereal grains.

When I interview new clients and they tell me they've already upped their fiber uptake, this is usually the kind of fiber they're talking about. I like to call them "water-phobe" fibers. I also refer to insoluble fibers as sweepers because they make their way through our digestive systems like a broom. They remain intact and pick up other foods along the way (while making the stool softer and bulkier). Everyone likes a thorough "clean out" to feel thin and flat-tummied.

Sweepers are an important component of healthy diets, but they cannot be your sole source of fiber. Clients often find it easy to eat more sweepers because they come in easy-access forms, like bran flakes, bran crackers, wheat crackers, and whole wheat bread. Simply adding these foods to your diet will surely send you to the bathroom. They will combat constipation and may increase regularity, both of which are great results. But will they fill you up and keep you satisfied?

Personally, I've never found a lunch of a bran cracker with butter spray all that satisfying. Stressing insoluble fiber while ignoring soluble fiber isn't sustainable, and it only gets you halfway there. You can eat all the nutrition bars or fiber-enriched yogurts you want, and down Metamucil like it's going out of style, but these habits won't promote weight loss, especially if the fiber is just an added ingredient in what is otherwise a high-calorie, high-sugar product. The only substantial weight-loss results I've seen in more than 10 years as a nutritionist comes from eating real, whole, hydrophilic foods.

Soluble Fiber: Sponges and Water-Loving Hydrophilics

Think about a kitchen sponge. You know the one—the dry, hard sponge that sits on the top corner of your sink. Place it under running water and it's instantly revitalized. It's filled up and ready to use, and all from a little water. The hydrophilic foods introduced in this plan will have the same effect on you.

When we ingest soluble fibers, they dissolve and form a gel in our intestines. This gel is the key to:

- **Steadying blood sugar and thus diminishing cravings.** The gel created by high-hydrophilic foods improves the way your body processes carbohydrates, and it decreases insulin response by slowing down glucose absorption. Have you ever longed for a vending machine pick-me-up only an hour after your morning bowl of Lucky Charms? This is because your breakfast lacked hydrophilic fiber. When you ingest foods with soluble fiber, it stops nasty cravings by keeping blood sugar levels steady.

- **Keeping you feeling full.** Hunger is the enemy when you're trying to lose weight (as I will discuss in subsequent chapters).

- **Maintaining digestive health.** When your digestive system is working optimally, your body responds by absorbing and burning the foods you eat more efficiently, which makes you lose weight more easily. The fiber gel helps food absorb your digestive juices and keeps your digestive mucosa in good condition. Here is one analogy I like to use with clients: If you saw patches of dry skin on your face, you'd buy creams to give your skin the moisture it's lacking; well, just as your face needs moisture, your digestive system also needs it to function correctly.

Gel-forming hydrophilic fibers can be split into two categories: pectin and mucilage.

Pectin is a complex carbohydrate found both in the cell walls of plants and between those cell walls, where it helps to regulate the flow of water to and from cells. Foods that are high in pectin include pears, apples, oranges, apricots, carrots, and beans.

In cooking, pectin is used as a natural thickening agent (because it gels!). In the body, pectin acts as a detoxifier, a gastrointestinal tract regulator, and an immune system stimulant. It also contains compounds that protect against ulcers and kidney injury. Pectin helps prevent a surge in blood glucose levels by promoting satiety and possibly by reducing the rate of glucose uptake following the consumption of glycemic carbohydrates, so it is good for people with diabetes. It also has been suggested that pectin can reduce heart disease and gallstones.

Several studies have reported a significant decrease in serum cholesterol (the total amount of cholesterol in your blood) and LDL (bad) cholesterol and an increase or no change in HDL (good) cholesterol in people taking pectin supplements. This cholesterol-lowering benefit may be a result of pectin's role in increasing the excretion of fecal cholesterol, fecal fat, sterols, or bile acids.

The first pectin available for purchase was derived from apples, which have a high amount of it. The properties of pectin were first identified by the French chemist and pharmacist Henri Braconnot, and his discovery soon led to pectin manufacturers making deals with apple juice makers for the remains of pressed apples.

Mucilage is really just a fancy word for slime. Remember the movie *Ghostbusters*, where the goal was *not* to be slimed by ghosts? Well, in the HD plan, slime is good.

Mucilage is a thick, gluey substance produced by nearly all plants. It is created by large polysaccharides (sugars) that form a semisoluble, viscous fiber in water. In plants, mucilage helps with holding water, storing food, and germinating seeds; it also serves as a membrane thickener and stabilizer. So foods high in mucilage are—you guessed it—hydrophilic!

> The plants commonly known as soapworts have so much mucilage they were used as soap. Early American colonists and pioneers used the sudsy plant to clean everything from homemade lace to pewter cups. And it was used for generations by farmers' wives on washday. Today, soapwort is still used as a "natural" soap and to clean delicate fabrics.

There are many mucilaginous herbs and foods that you can add to your diet to help promote a leaner, healthier you. They play an important role in immunity support, mainly by helping to hydrate the mucosal cells that line your mouth, eyes, nose, throat, and intestines. Some mucilaginous herbs are aloe, arnica, nettle, sage, basil, slippery elm, and parsley. Familiar mucilaginous foods are okra, figs, green beans, chia seeds, and seaweeds (like agar and kelp).

TOP 10 HYDROPHILIC FOODS

The extensive HD plan food lists are provided in Chapter 5 along with a detailed outline of your 12-week journey into forever living in HD. However, I wanted to share with you now some favorites that have been staples in my practice. These foods *love* water, and I love them for it! While the HD plan will introduce you to many new foods and how to prepare and incorporate them into your diet, here are my top 10!

1. CHIA SEEDS

Often I am asked how I began to explore the hydrophilic properties of different foods. The answer is, it was my dad who started me on this expedition, and it started with chia. My dad has a thirst for knowledge. He wants to know everything. As a kid, I found it very annoying to have a dad who was always quizzing us on the facts and history of everything! But as an adult, I came to appreciate his resourcefulness.

While attending a lecture with my sister (who's an architect) on upcoming materials with unique properties, my dad stumbled upon a demonstration of a nanofiber cloth that was paper-thin but swelled up like a sponge when placed in water. The exhibitors explained that the material was hydrophilic. Curious as always, my dad wondered if there were foods with this same quality because he had heard me complaining that hunger is often what derails my clients from reaching their weight goals. What if a hydrophilic food could keep hunger pangs at bay by filling you up?

That's when he came across the chia seed—a small black or white seed with the capacity to absorb water up to 12 times its weight! He told me to research it, and unlike my younger self, I was open to his suggestion. Yes, these are the same seeds used for the infamous Chia Pet clay

20 WAYS TO USE HYDRO-BOOSTING CHIA SEEDS

1. Mix into morning oatmeal or healthy cereal.
2. Mix into yogurt.
3. Add to shakes and smoothies.
4. Add to soups to thicken the stock.
5. Add to gravies to thicken.
6. Use as an egg substitute: 1 tablespoon chia seeds with ¼ cup water for 1 egg.
7. Grind seeds and add them to warm almond milk.
8. Make a pudding with a tapioca consistency (see recipe on page 221).
9. Add to beaten eggs, soak for 10 minutes, and make a chia omelet or chia scramble.
10. Sprinkle over a salad.
11. Soak in almond milk and add the mixture to a broccoli, cauliflower, sweet potato, or turnip mash.
12. Add to dips and spreads.
13. Stir in while cooking beans.
14. Stir in while cooking grains.
15. Toss into a stir-fry.
16. Grind seeds and mix with ground meat for burgers, meatballs, or meat loaf.
17. Add to canned salmon or tuna.
18. Add to salad dressings.
19. Toast (for a nuttier flavor) and sprinkle over vegetables and salads.
20. Make Chia Gel. (I love to keep this in the fridge. You will be surprised how many times you can use it to "boost" your meals. See page 158 for the recipe.)

figures. But chia seeds are not just for fun anymore; now they're for breakfast. They're a "hydro-boosting" food and a critical element of the HD plan because of their ability to encourage satiety and because of their nutritional value.

Chia (*Salvia hispanica*) is a member of the Lamiaceae (mint) family. The genus name *Salvia* is derived from the Latin word meaning "to save." The common name *chia* derives from the Mayan word for "strengthening." Chia seeds were domesticated in Mexico as early as 2700 BC and were a staple food of the Mayans and Aztecs. They were so valued that they were even used as a form of currency. Chia seeds were also known for their medicinal properties and used topically to help heal wounds. Aztec warriors reputedly survived on chia seeds during their conquests on the battlefield—and at home; apparently, chia seeds were eaten to enhance one's sex life. Considered an energy tonic, they were used in other high-endurance activities as well, such as long-distance running.

When I began researching chia seeds, I discovered that these ancient conceptions of their health benefits hold up to 21st-century scrutiny. And since they absorb up to 12 times their weight in water in under 10 minutes, they are filling as well. Chia's ability to hold on to water also means you maintain hydration and retain electrolytes. And when your body is properly hydrated, nutrients from the foods you ingest are absorbed more efficiently. Since chia seeds swell in volume when mixed with liquid and have no discernible flavor, they can bulk up your favorite snacks and meals, displacing calories without compromising taste! This chia capability will be discussed further in Chapter 10's section on how to make Chia Gel.

If all that doesn't make it a superfood already, these little seeds also contain:

- Eight times more omega-3s than salmon
- 30 percent more antioxidants than blueberries
- 25 percent more fiber than flax
- Three times more iron than spinach
- 15 times more magnesium than broccoli
- Six times more calcium than milk
- Two times more potassium than a banana

2. OKRA

Okra is a fantastic vegetable that I revere for its slime factor! It is known for being high in hydrophilic (soluble) fiber due to its great mucilage content. I don't think we use okra enough. It is a low-calorie food, too—36 calories per cooked cup.

Many people shy away from okra because of its slimy consistency, but it's easy to alleviate the goo factor when you add okra to stews, soups, and stir-fries. Okra is high in vitamins A, B_6, and C; folate; calcium; iron; and magnesium. When okra is added to your meals, you won't be hungry for hours.

3. OATMEAL

This happens to be a favorite of many nutrition enthusiasts. It is absolutely my number-one choice for breakfast because of its ability to HD satiate. Add chia seeds to oatmeal and there is no better way to start your day!

Oatmeal is a perfect example of an HD food because you can see the gelling process before your very eyes while cooking it (although you can eat oatmeal raw for the same benefits!). Nevertheless, all my clients have an extreme reaction to oatmeal: They either love it or would rather eat wallpaper paste. Perhaps it's a texture issue. Or it may be a "block" food (which I discuss further in the "Beware of the Block Food" sidebar). In any event, if you're one of the haters, I urge you to reconsider oatmeal. If you still hate it, don't worry. Other options abound. I just had to make that plea.

If you love oatmeal, however, you will be happy to hear that in addition to soluble fiber, oatmeal has 6 grams of protein per serving. It also contains the minerals phosphorus, potassium, selenium, manganese, and some iron.

A 15-year study published in the *American Journal of Lifestyle Medicine* found that oatmeal—thanks to a type of polysaccharide called beta-glucan—lowers cholesterol and decreases the risk of heart disease. Specifically, oatmeal was shown to reduce serum (total) cholesterol and LDL (bad) cholesterol while not changing levels of HDL (good) cholesterol.[3]

But which oats do you buy? This is a common concern among my clients who want to make oatmeal a staple in their diet. There are three types of oats on the market—steel-cut, rolled (old fashioned), and quick (instant). Which one do you choose? Steel-cut oats are the least processed and require the most cooking time. Old-fashioned oats are steam-processed and rolled into oats that stay fresh for longer periods, with a cooking time of between 5 and 10 minutes. Quick or instant oat flakes have been steamed longer and flattened more than rolled oats, so they cook the fastest.

In the USDA's nutrient database, all of the different types of oats show the same nutritional profile. The difference, however, is in how they are digested. Instant oats digest the fastest since they are processed to cook quickly. And when a food digests quicker, it does not keep you as full.

Therefore, I suggest you go for rolled since some steel-cut oats take around 40 minutes to cook. I want you to actually have the oatmeal, not stress about preparation. You may love to cook, in which case go for the steel-cut, but my experience has been that if it takes more than 10 minutes, it's not happening. I have recipes in Chapter 11 that use rolled oats and even instant for those crazy, hectic days. Instant is fine to use if you prep it the HD way, with no added sugars and with the addition of hydro-boosting chia seeds (to keep you satiated longer). So don't stress!

4. PEARS

I encourage my clients to eat fruits. Lots of them. I particularly stress the high-hydrophilic fruits that contain pectin. We have all heard an apple a day keeps the doctor away; well, so does a pear. Pears actually have *more* pectin than apples. And like other high-hydrophilic foods, they help with digestion, lowering your cholesterol and regulating your body's absorption of sugar. Not to mention this delicious snack will keep you HD satiated.

When you eat the fiber-rich skin along with the flesh, you're even better off. The skin contains the antioxidant quercetin, which prevents cancer and artery damage that can lead to heart problems. A recent study at Cornell University found quercetin also protects against Alzheimer's disease. Pears are less likely to produce an adverse or allergic response than other fruits. (Pears are often recommended as a safe fruit to introduce to infants.)

Look for my Poached Cinnamon Pears recipe on page 232. But the beauty of the pear is you can simply pack it in your bag and go—no prep required.

5. BARLEY

Barley is a fantastic hydrophilic grain, with an exceptional capacity to absorb water. It also has a delicious nutty flavor and pastalike texture, which is why it is one of my favorite grains to add to salads, soups, and side dishes. It's even good to swap for oatmeal in the morning for a change. In the store, you'll find hulled, pearled, and pot barley. Go for the pot barley. It's between hulled and pearled in terms of how much it's been processed. And it retains its nutritive punch while being the easiest to work with.

6. BRUSSELS SPROUTS

I admit it: I can eat Brussels sprouts as a snack, with my lunch, and with my dinner every day. My enthusiasm for these mini cabbages hasn't

BEWARE OF THE BLOCK FOOD

People *love* to talk to me about their food likes and dislikes. I don't mean just my clients, but friends and family members, too. I have a distinct memory of my husband, Jonathan, telling me he hated nuts when we first met. He was so adamant about it! I couldn't get him to eat a nut if I begged. Even my parents knew not to offer any nuts to Jonathan. As the years went by and my eating habits infiltrated more of our snacks and meals, Jonathan ingested some almonds. And you know what? He liked them! Now I can't stop him from eating nuts. He eats them constantly—all sorts of nuts. In fact, sometimes he eats too much.

For whatever reason, nuts were my husband's "block" food.

When he started to eat nuts, my mom caught on and started buying them for when we came to visit. My mom loves to feed all my boys, all the time. One day in excitement, my mom said, "Jonathan, I'm roasting your nuts, and they're delicious." My boys laughed for days over that line.

I have found block foods to be an issue for so many clients. Oatmeal is a big one. Other times it is certain vegetables, fruits, or fish, and the list goes on. Often I will say, "Give it a try and see if you like it. It certainly isn't a have-to, but you may have a block." Many times I'm right, and this block food becomes a favorite on the HD plan. No joke. Big takeaway: Try new things even if you think you'll hate them.

impressed my eldest son, who rolls his eyes when I proclaim, "Mmmm, like candy!" and beg him to try one. Some clients have the same reaction to my Brussels passion. But it's for real: I love them. Plus they contain enough hydrophilic fiber to keep you full for hours.

Brussels sprouts are part of the cruciferous vegetable family (cabbages), and the American Cancer Society includes them as a key dietary recommendation. The cancer protection we get from Brussels sprouts is largely related to four specific glucosinolates: glucoraphanin, glucobrassicin, sinigrin, and gluconasturtiin. All cruciferous vegetables contain glucosinolates, and these phytonutrients are important for our health because they are the chemical starting points for a variety of cancer-protective substances. In short, cruciferous vegetables detoxify. Lab studies show that one of the phytochemicals found in cruciferous vegetables—sulforaphane—can stimulate enzymes in the body that detoxify carcinogens before they damage cells.

Be sure not to overcook your Brussels sprouts though. This will cause them to not only lose nutritional value and taste but also emit an odor like that of rotten eggs (because the overcooking causes chemicals in the sprouts to produce sulfur). Steaming them for 6 to 8 minutes is all you need. Oven roasted and sautéed Brussels are terrific, too.

7. KIDNEY BEANS

The truth of the matter is that *all* beans are high-hydrophilic foods. I picked kidney beans because I love them in chili-like soups, and they are almost always an option at make-it-yourself salad bars. (By the way, I will teach you how to build a perfect HD salad that keeps you full for hours.)

One of the points I stress to clients is that you can choose beans as your protein in a salad to replace the usual chicken, turkey, or tuna fish. When doing so, the portion is hefty (1 cup) and very satisfying. I will explain further how to incorporate these important hydrophilic superfoods into your diet later on. I find that clients who begin to include more bean-focused meals in their diets love the variety and get amazing HD results. Red beans, like kidney beans, also have a very high antioxidant value.

8. CHICKPEAS

Here is another salad bar favorite and my bean of choice for meals and snacks on the HD plan. Chickpeas are high in hydrophilic (soluble) fiber and keep you full for hours. I love grabbing some HD crudité veggies along with ½ cup Roasted Chickpeas (page 231) or chickpea spread in the afternoon. It keeps you satiated all the way to dinner. (Ever notice how chickpeas have bumps? Most other beans are smooth. If you look closely, these bumps resemble a chick's beak. That's why they are called chickpeas.)

Eating more beans is proven to decrease the risk of coronary disease. In a study of almost 10,000 men and women in the United States, participants who ate beans more than four times a week had a 22 percent lower risk of coronary heart disease and an 11 percent lower risk of cardiovascular events than those who ate beans less than once a week.[4]

9. ORANGES

I have great childhood memories of drinking OJ at breakfast like my morning cup of coffee. With every sip, I felt like I was fighting infections and getting strong. Oranges have always been recognized for being an excellent source of vitamin C and they are, providing 53.2 milligrams per 100 grams, which is about 90 percent of the Recommended Dietary Allowance.

However, as I became more educated in nutrition, I realized I had to stop downing the juice and start eating the whole fruit. Whole oranges are chock-full of hydrophilic fiber. They contain a lot of belly-filling pectin. I cannot say the same for my once-treasured OJ.

I love oranges as a between-meals snack with pistachios or almonds. I now want to make a plea: Do not peel away the thick, white outer layer that comes off in strings and dump it in the compost pile. It is quite a tedious task and totally unnecessary! This layer is called the pith, and it's part of the reason why the orange is so wonderful. The pith contains a lot of the pectin in addition to nearly the same amount of vitamin C as the flesh. So save yourself time and effort, and just eat it.

Oranges are also a wonderful source of phytochemicals, vitamin A, B-complex vitamins, potassium, and calcium. So grab an orange on the HD plan and enjoy.

10. AGAR

I discovered agar because it was a food that fit the HD plan criteria. Sometimes referred to as agar-agar or kanten, it is a gelling agent made from seaweed and widely used in Southeast Asia. Agar is 80 percent hydrophilic fiber (just add water and the flakes swell up into a thick gel). It has no calories, no carbs, no sugar, no fat—just fiber. Its hydrophilic fiber reabsorbs glucose in the stomach, passes through the digestive system quickly, and inhibits the body from retaining and storing excess fat. Its water-absorbing properties also aid in waste elimination. Agar absorbs bile, and by doing so, it causes the body to dissolve more cholesterol.

Agar has also been reported to help suppress appetite and aid in weight loss. A 2005 study based in Japan and published in *Diabetes, Obesity and Metabolism* compared two groups of participants who were overweight and had type 2 diabetes. One group was placed on a regular diet and the other on a kanten-supplemented diet for 12 weeks. The study claimed the kanten-supplemented group lost more weight and had lower fasting glucose levels, lower blood pressure, and lower cholesterol than the nonkanten group.[5]

It took me awhile to find a way to use agar, but I did and now I love it. I want you to become familiar with it on your HD journey because it is an amazing hydrophilic culinary ingredient that can help satisfy that afternoon or after-dinner sweets craving. You can use agar to make delicious pudding that rivals the processed brands found in the supermarket. It's easy to make and it's "free" on the HD plan, tallying up less than 50 calories a serving! Check out the recipe on page 220.

Okay, I know I said top 10, but there's actually one more food I have to include! Nori (dried seaweed) is used to wrap sushi. Nori is around 35 percent fiber by weight, and most of it is hydrophilic. It is sold in thin, flat sheets at health food stores. I love all seaweeds, but nori is my top pick because on the HD plan it can replace a "bread" and I consider it a "carb fake-out" food. Check out the Nori Vegetable Wrap on page 227.

Now you can see how the HD plan foods can keep you full, vibrant, and healthy. In 12 weeks you will completely revolutionize the way you build your meals, and you will learn to live in HD in the process. Are you ready?

ILANA, 21,
Lost 28 Pounds

Before HD: Even in middle school, I remember not feeling too great about my body. I was always thinking, "Why can't I be skinny?" So I tried some really extreme diets. I tried high protein and no carbs. That just killed my energy levels. I tried cutting my calories really, really low. That worked for a while—with really quick results—and then my weight bounced back the minute I started eating more. I was really unhealthy. I even remember trying Hydroxycut at one point. I stopped using it because it just wasn't making me feel good; my heart raced on it. My first year of college, I just kept gaining weight, and I didn't realize it until I came home and was 153 pounds.

Starting strong: The first thing Keren and I tackled was the mental stuff. Like, what do you want to change? Why do you want to change it? So I made a commitment and signed the contract.

New foods: I love drinking lemon water in the morning. It's so fresh and really wakes you up. For breakfast I have oatmeal with chia seeds. And I eat raw carrots, jicama, and celery with bean dip almost every day. I love broccoli, and I started eating more fruits, like apples, oranges, and berries. I also love big, fresh salads built the way Keren taught me.

Never misses: I was really into frozen yogurt at one point. I'd have it with my friends all the time. My goal was to cut it down to just once a week. Then, all of a sudden, every time I would have frozen yogurt, I felt like it was kind of nasty and I wasn't benefiting from eating it anymore. So just cutting it out for a while helped me acknowledge that it wasn't good for me. My body was naturally realizing that it wasn't getting the nutrition it needed from the frozen yogurt.

Ilana really took control of her IFs (see page 84 and Chapter 7). Once she got a handle on them, it became easier to see the big picture. She quickly discovered that the temporary enjoyment she would experience when she ate certain foods wasn't worth it. And she approaches her diet in an entirely new manner now.

Unexpected bonus: I naturally stopped eating meat because I increased my intake of vegetables and fruits.

Lesson learned: When you eat a lot, you stretch your stomach, and if you stretch it too much, you never get that full feeling. So I eat small meals every few hours. I don't like eating big meals because I feel so full—and gross—afterward.

New mantra: Think about how food is affecting your body. Like, "What is pizza going to add to my nutrition?" Your body is hungry for nutrients, so give it nutrients.

Sustaining in HD: I started feeling better about myself, and people started noticing. People pick up on that stuff. I was glowing inside and out, and it just felt really nice. Finally, I was finding my inner confidence.

Inspiring words: Anybody can do this. You just need to be motivated. You also need to look past immediate results and really concentrate on making this plan a part of your everyday life. It's not about being skinny. It's about being a healthy person inside and out, being in tune with your body, and being in tune with yourself.

2

DECIDING TO LIVE IN **HD**

"The most difficult thing is the decision to act; the rest is merely tenacity. The fears are paper tigers. You can do anything you decide to do. You can act to change and control your life and the procedure. The process is its own reward."

—AMELIA EARHART

Every time I begin a new journey with a client, we start by talking about what brought that client through my door. Here are some things I have heard over the years.

"I'm 40 pounds heavier than I was 10 years ago. I want to get rid of it, once and for all."

"This extra roll on my stomach has got to go."

"I want to look as good as the women in that Gap commercial."

"I want to look like I did before my kids were born."

Now, let's say your goal is to learn how to play the guitar. (This is probably not what you were expecting to read in a weight-loss book, but it's an example I use with my clients all the time.) What do you want? You want to be able to pick up a guitar and jam at a party. (In my daydream, it's Santana's "Black Magic Woman," but you can choose your own song.) And then one day, down the road, you are at a party and you casually pick up a guitar that's laying around, and the next thing you know, everyone is looking at you in awe because you are just *that* good.

And sure, you made it *look* easy. But in order to get that appreciative applause (and envious stares), you had to start by learning the basics. You endured tedious weeks of training your fingers to play the chords. You had to *decide*, over and over again, to sacrifice a chunk of time each day to practice your scales, which likely wasn't all that much fun (maybe even boring) and certainly wasn't immediately rewarding. Nobody was staring at you in awe then, right? But you honored your commitment to yourself and eventually you were playing "Twinkle, Twinkle, Little Star" and then "Happy Birthday" and then "Over the Rainbow."

And you *kept* practicing. You made daily *decisions* to not click on the television but to pick up the guitar instead. Getting better took several small decisions, and some days making those decisions was much harder than others. Those *Real Housewives* can be mighty enticing, after all. But it happened: You were able to jam and look darn cool doing it. And it was *totally* worth it—not only for the looks on everyone's faces, but also for the pure joy of accomplishing something that required dedication. Whoever else you are, you're now someone who plays the guitar.

We are going to explore your food decisions throughout the HD journey, but right now I want you to think about all of your accomplishments. What are they? Is it your relationship with your spouse? Your thriving career? Or is it your wonderful, well-disciplined children? Is it that you graduated from an Ivy League school? Whatever you love and admire about yourself, chances are you made sacrifices to get it.

I only remind you of this because when it comes to losing weight, we tend to want quick fixes—a pill, a fad, or a powder to sprinkle on mac-and-cheese that renders it magically calorie free. But if you want to become the CEO of a Fortune 500 company, do you swallow a pill and—poof!—become a CEO overnight?

Of course not. If you are a parent, I know you get this. Your very smart, capable kid comes home with a C and you ask him, "How did this happen? Didn't you study?" He responds, "No, I understood it in class. I didn't think I had to study." So you start rambling about how "you get out of life what you put into it" and that you'd be fine with the C if he had tried his hardest. You remind him that getting the A means no video chats, no texts, and a lot of sitting in silence with a book—sacrifices, in other words. (Excuse my ranting, but this is a speech I am used to giving at my house.)

But here is the point of all these analogies: The first step in the HD plan starts with the exact same kind of daily decision making. Everybody who wants to get fit has to make daily decisions, no matter who that person may be. Think of some celebrities whose hot bodies you're envious of. Guess what? They work at those abs and taut triceps, especially if they are—like so many of us—over 30, raising kids, and juggling busy schedules! Sure, they may have chefs cooking their meals and trainers telling them how to move, but *they* are ultimately doing the work. *They're* deciding for themselves what to put in their mouths; they're deciding to work out rather than go shopping or flashing their privates to the paparazzi or whatever else celebrities do with their free time.

I always refer to James O. Prochaska and Carlo DiClemente's Stages of Change model to illustrate that the HD journey is a slow climb. Prochaska and DiClemente worked together in the psychology department at the University of Rhode Island in the 1980s, and their model demonstrates that when people decide to make life-altering changes, process is everything. Whether the goal is quitting smoking or learning Pilates, one must progress through five different stages before a new habit is fully formed. These five stages are precontemplation, contemplation, preparation, action, and maintenance.

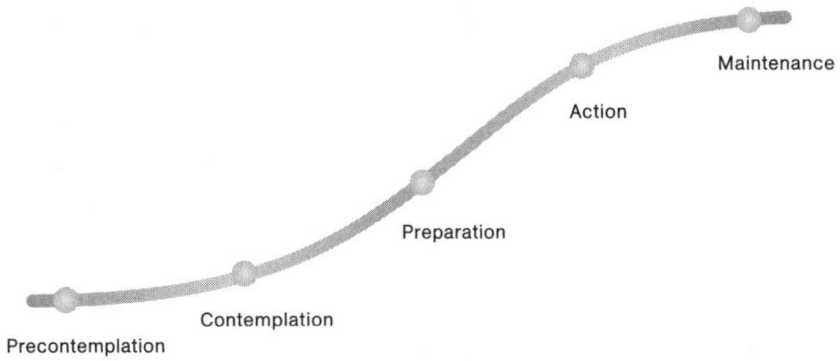

- ***Precontemplation (not ready).*** People at this stage aren't planning on changing and may not have accepted that change might be good for them. For these people, change is at least 6 months away. They may not even *know* they need to make changes in their lives. But they're learning more every day, whether by listening to the news or hearing about the weight-loss success of a friend or family member, and they are starting to imagine how a different, more positive future is possible. Still, two big obstacles stand in their way: (1) they consistently *over*estimate the negative side of change, and (2) they lowball the benefits of it.

- ***Contemplation (getting ready).*** People at this stage are starting to see how their habits and decisions may be causing them trouble. They have made a decision: They *will* change—someday. But why the wait? Well, they know more about the pros of change, but their list of cons is still long. Whether it's because the climb ahead seems too steep or because of uncertainty about having the right support structures in place, they're not taking action just yet. At this stage, encouraging friends can make a huge difference.
- ***Preparation (readiness).*** Here people are gearing up to make changes to their daily routines within the next 30 days. They may already be taking small steps. Simply announcing their intentions to friends and family can be one such step because it starts to build an accountability network. Most importantly, their thoughts and daydreams are focused not on how hard the climb will be but on how terrific they'll feel once they reach the top.
- ***Action.*** People at this stage are in a groove. They are working and need to keep working. The temptation to backslide is there, but overall their commitment to change is being renewed almost daily. It's important for people at this stage to continue to explore new substitute activities for past unhealthy behaviors, congratulate themselves on progress made, and steer clear of some situations—and people!—that could sabotage their efforts.
- ***Maintenance (sustaining action).*** New habits aren't so new anymore and are practically the "new normal." At this point, what was once a new behavior, habit, or lifestyle is at least 6 months old. In stressful situations, there is still the potential to backslide, but generally these people are feeling and experiencing that change is good.

This is a climb! But by picking up this book, by reading this section, you're already halfway up the hill. You will not run to the top in 1 week, but if you are committed and trust the process, you *will* get there.

Whenever I meet new clients, I explain this to them as well: When you have flipped the switch to do the work, you are halfway there. I explain that every week, for no fewer than 12 weeks, we will prepare and take action together, back and forth, until the top is reached. Please also know that once you reach your desired weight, you must continue to make decisions. Even a rock star doesn't stow away her guitar once she's gotten really good at playing "Black Magic Woman." She picks up that guitar for fun and profit and embraces it. And whether you can feel it now or not, I promise you that after 12 weeks of living in HD, you'll retain the concepts you acquired along the way. You'll still need to "practice" them, but they'll absolutely be easier to do.

I am here to be your advocate. This book is your route map, but please do not forget that *you* are making the journey. I cannot give you the tools of discipline and passion. Fighting the twin temptations of complacency and overconfidence is a solo battle and often a tough emotional one. I *will* make it easier, though.

This is an interesting first step because I haven't even started talking about eating yet! But deciding is a necessary and crucial phase. You have to *make the decision* that this is what you want, that you deserve this, and that you will put in the effort to achieve it.

Ever hear the expression, "I am climbing the ladder in my career"? Well, now you are climbing the ladder for your health and your body. It is hard work, but the rewards are phenomenal! Have you decided to live your life in HD? If the answer is a resounding YES, then please turn the page.

CHERYL, 56,
Lost 25 Pounds

Before HD: I went to the doctor and I got a terrible report. She said, "Your sugars are very close to being diabetic." And my cholesterol wasn't great either. I was never a very big eater, I was having wine every night, salad dressing on all of my salads, and half an avocado every day. I was also having cappuccinos at the end of dinner, and so on. So all of these extra things added up to a lot of weight gained over the years.

Starting strong: I never really ate fish, and I started eating salmon and branzino on the HD plan. And now they're my favorites. I always remember to include the high-hydrophilic vegetables Keren stresses in all of my meals.

New foods: Peanut butter from Whole Foods; there's no added anything. It's amazing and it's filling. I have 1 tablespoon on a Decision Nutrition Chia Bagel, or in the afternoon, I have 1 tablespoon on an apple.

Never misses: I haven't had a piece of chocolate or cake or bread. But I'm not really craving anything I shouldn't have.

Unexpected bonus: My husband is eating a little bit better, too. Not perfectly—he's a big eater—but now I order salmon for both of us. A year ago, he would have never touched it.

Lesson learned: Steamed vegetables are delicious!

New mantra: It's not really a diet. It's more like a way of life.

Sustaining in HD: You have to plan. Otherwise, you're not going to eat when—or what—you should.

Inspiring words: I never feel like I'm hungry, and I look like a whole different person.

3

DAILY HD DECISIONS— UNCOVERING YOUR CURRENT HABITS

"I have come to believe that caring for myself is not self-indulgent. Caring for myself is an act of survival."

—AUDRE LORDE

Before I make you sign the HD oath in blood (just kidding, sort of), let's take a look at where the food decisions you make each day might be a little out of focus. Everyone's journey to HD is different—and if someone wants to just start the HD eating plan right away, that's fine—but to really help ensure long-term weight-loss success, it's good to first get insight into the issues you are confronting on a daily basis.

How do you begin to explore your current habits?

Once I have thoroughly reviewed the importance of making the decision to live in HD with a client, the next step involves a comprehensive investigation of that person's "pre-HD" daily food lifestyle. It is important to understand how someone approaches food decisions presently in order to uncover what issues need to be addressed going forward.

3-DAY DIET RECALL

To get insight into a client's food history, I have that person perform a 3-day diet recall, which is basically a food report of 3 random days of the week (I recommend 2 weekdays and 1 weekend day). I discuss the importance of food logging during your HD journey in Chapter 4, but this is different. The point of a 3-day diet recall is to reveal present habits that could be interfering with your weight goal. I like to call these bad habits "health derailers."

To start your investigation, you will need three food log sheets, which you can find on page 240 or at my Web site, decisionnutrition.com. Then pick the days you would like to examine. Of course, every day is different, but we all have our habits. As you take your recall and read the client stories in this chapter, you will discover your own.

Keep in mind, tracking calories is not really the concern here. As you do your 3-day diet recall, I want you to pay attention to these three things: (1) what you eat, (2) how much you eat, and (3) how you feel when you eat. "What" and "how much" are obvious concerns, but paying attention to "when" you eat is also very important. Say you skip breakfast to save on calories, but then find yourself feeling woozy and cranky come 11:00 a.m.; in this state, you are unlikely to make good portion choices.

Before embarking on your diet recall, become familiar with the following Hunger Determination Scale, which contains numbered descriptions of various degrees of "hunger," or lack thereof. You will refer to the scale before and after all of your meals and snacks. This is a process I call "collecting your hunger data."

The Hunger Determination Scale is a very important tool for living in HD because it helps you tune in to *your* body signals. We tend to take care of others in our lives—partners, spouses, friends, children—and be in tune with their desires. But we often forget to pay attention to our own needs. When you start recording your hunger data, you are going to become more aware of what your body needs and what it doesn't need. And you will start to expose eating patterns that may be contributing to the "fuzz" and unwanted pounds.

I want you to take a few minutes to really contemplate the Hunger Determination Scale. Are there any numbers you relate to? It is important to know where you experience your most daunting moments. It is different for everyone, although there are common patterns.

Certainly, we all relate to these numbers in one way or another. There are days when I tend to my children in the morning, go to work, and by the time I look up at the clock it's already 2:30 p.m. and I am a solid 2.

HUNGER DETERMINATION SCALE

1. This is the smallest number on the scale; it means there is no food in your stomach and you are famished! You would eat the kitchen table if you could. You are irritable and have a headache.
2. Your stomach is making loud grumbles; everyone can hear you're hungry. You are irritable and tired, and the kitchen table still looks mighty enticing.
3. You are getting uncomfortably hungry. Your stomach is starting to stir. You watch the clock because you need to eat a meal fast (or you will go down to a 2).
4. You are slightly hungry, but a small snack will do.
5. You are in neutral: not hungry and not full. This is how you should feel after a suitable HD snack. When you are "feeling like a 5," food is not a distraction.
6. You are nearly satisfied. Food is not seducing you, but a few more bites seem to be in order.
7. You are HD satiated. This is the term I use to describe the feeling you get after eating a meal using the HD principles and you walk away very content but not stuffed. You are "good to go" for many hours.
8. You took one bite too many. Your pants are tight.
9. Your pants are getting tighter. You need to unbutton them at this point.
10. This is the largest number on the scale; it means your stomach is extremely full. You ate way too much. You are nauseated. In fact, you are going to throw up.

READING YOUR HD NUMBERS

1, 2, and 3 = metabolism abuse (and binge alert!) = weight gain

4 = be prepared with an HD snack or you'll head back to a 1, 2, or 3

5, 6, and 7 = good numbers to aim for (7 being ideal)

8, 9, and 10 = mindless eating = weight gain

And, yes, at that point I could gobble down my desk! There have also been too many Thanksgiving dinners where I regrettably have experienced a 10.

I always begin the hunger data portion of a client's assessment by discussing the consequences of the lower half of the Hunger Determination Scale. If you experience a 1, 2, or 3 during the day, three major concerns emerge. The first is that your ravenous self will make bad food decisions when you finally decide to eat. It is very difficult to sit down to dinner with friends when you are at a 2 and not devour the entire bread basket, even though your brain knows it's not the best decision. (By the way, don't ever go on a date at a 1, 2, or 3!) The second concern regarding the "when" of eating is that if you dip below a 4 on the scale two or three times a day, you *will* have trouble losing weight. You will most likely overeat because your stomach is screaming to be filled. I always stress this point because even good foods become less good once portion sizes swell up. (Of course, the worst combo is making bad food selections *and* overindulging.) I will review portions in Chapter 6.

The third concern is that if you experience a 1, 2, or 3 during the day, most likely you have not eaten for many hours. So many people skip breakfast. But when you run out the door without breakfast and continue with your day, your body suffers consequences. Essentially, you have fasted all through the night and morning and by lunchtime your body is in a state of confusion. It was hoping for food, but for some reason you're holding out on it.

Your body is an amazing machine. At the 1, 2, or 3 stages, it will begin to slow down to preserve energy. Your body doesn't know what your eating plans are; it just knows that it is not being nourished. *You* may know that in 2 hours you'll be seated at an extravagant luncheon, but your body doesn't! So it is going to start holding on to what it's got. And when you do sit down for that meal, it will hold on to that, too. Even when you exhibit fabulous willpower by eating a perfectly portioned salad, your body will not process this meal as well as it would if it was running more efficiently. Your body is going to hold on to that salad for dear life because another food shortage may be just around the corner. That beautiful salad will not be metabolized properly and will get stored as fat! This is a common phenomenon, and it is abusive to your body and your metabolism. (And, most likely, you are not having a perfect salad anyway because bad food decisions are common when you are at a low number on the scale!)

The middle section of the scale—4, 5, 6, and 7—are the numbers that I want my clients to become really familiar with on their HD journey. These numbers feel good! You feel grounded and in control and are able to concentrate on whatever you have to do. Think of 4 as your body sending you a message: "When was the last time I ate? When am I eating again, and should I maybe have an apple and 10 almonds now to tide me over?" At a 7, you've most likely just eaten a satisfying (but not huge) meal, and you won't even be thinking about food for the next 3 hours.

And, yes, we all know the numbers 8, 9, or 10. We have all eaten past the stage of feeling comfortable, and we've all eaten when not actually physiologically hungry. There are so many ways we can numb ourselves to our bodies' signals. Reasons for eating when not physiologically hungry include:

Peer pressure (you're out with friends, and it would be awkward—or boring—not to eat)

Out of habit, like eating in front of the TV or at the movies, just because that's what you always do

Using food as a reward

Boredom

Relaxation

Anger

Happiness

Sadness

Celebratory (when the party begins, all mindfulness is out)

It is important to be aware of when you are mindlessly eating and to understand your own triggers.

The first step to using this scale is to just become aware of what numbers you relate to in a typical day. Mindless eating can be a hard habit to break, though, because much of it is related to bad habits or emotions. For example, if you always eat your dinner while catching up on Facebook, and blow past 7 without realizing it, a good rule would be to get on Facebook *after* your meal. Or if you find yourself stress-eating after the whole house is asleep, make a rule to not open the kitchen cabinet after 9:00 p.m. Take a bath or read a book instead. Or if you know that a Super Bowl party will tempt you to eat until you've reached a 10, have an HD plan!

Being conscious of your patterns and triggers is an important step to understanding your diet character. Once you get an idea of what yours is, you will be better able to address the health derailers getting in the way of your HD life. So what is a diet character, you ask?

A CAST OF DIET CHARACTERS

Well, there are many different personas, shapes, sizes, and ages that walk through the door of my practice. I sometimes think of my office as a movie set. Everyone who enters is a different character, but all of my "actors" have common goals: They want to feel better, and they want the number on the scale to drop. They have memorized an entire script of reasons why they have not been successful losing weight. They classify their dieting history in a neat little storyline and say, "This is me."

Here's the thing: You are not a character in a movie! Your life is not scripted, and you can change the course of your dieting history. I am going to share some "characters" that have walked into my office, plus a breakdown of the habits that were hindering their weight loss, so you can see if you may be typecasting yourself.

On-the-Go Gobbler

Theresa—a fiery redhead in her early forties with a big, demanding job—was lively and talked a mile a minute, and I was encouraged to see such energy right off the bat. But as we got deeper into the initial consultation, her outgoing personality deflated and the tears started rolling down her cheeks as she told me about the 30 extra pounds she had put on over the last 5 years. "I don't get it," said Theresa. "I've tried it all—Weight Watchers, Nutrisystem, you name it. I really make an effort. Yet I continually gain weight despite my efforts."

Theresa's breaking point was when she and her friends joined a Biggest Loser contest at her gym. The prize was $1,500, and she thought, "If this can't motivate me, what else can?" Theresa felt like she was trying hard, but she watched all of her friends lose weight while her scale stayed put.

Theresa—a "professional dieter"—was fed up with her lack of results.

She was desperate to take off the alarming amount of weight that had crept up on her, and she was feeling hopeless. "My body has changed with age," she told me. "I just can't lose." But that wasn't true. Though Theresa's perimenopausal stage of life might have been posing a challenge, her 3-day diet recall shed a lot of light on why the numbers on her scale wouldn't budge.

Always on the go, Theresa, who lived alone, would typically run out of the house hungry, forgoing breakfast because her refrigerator would always be empty. She'd grab a coffee en route to the office and—if she wasn't on a particular diet—sometimes she'd get an egg and cheese sandwich. But more often than not, Theresa would skip breakfast altogether, figuring she'd bank the calories for later. Lunch would be ordered in, and her selection would depend on what delivery joint her coworkers had chosen. She'd never snack between meals (again, she was saving her calories). And three or four times a week, Theresa would exercise; then she'd have a late dinner with friends or takeout.

Theresa's 3-day diet recall uncovered the following on-the-go health derailers. Remember, the danger zone is a 1, 2, or 3 on the Hunger Scale.

- **Skipping meals.** Being ravenous before a meal is counterproductive. When your body hasn't eaten for 6 hours, your metabolism slows because your body doesn't know you're going out to dinner!
- **Not paying attention to hunger signals.** Extreme hunger will cause you to make bad eating decisions because you'll be desperately craving food, any food.
- **Not having a stock of healthy foods ready.** This tends to make you susceptible to nibbling whatever is around or overordering high-fat, high-sodium, low-fiber fast foods or takeout.
- **Relying on fast-food meals and takeout.** Most foods not prepared by you have hidden calories and fats, are overprocessed, and are generally provided (and therefore eaten) in oversize portions—none of which are good for you.

Chubby Perpetual Exerciser

Remy—a mom of two older boys—was fed up with not being able to lose weight. Because her children were grown (one son was in high school, and the other was already in college) and didn't need her as much, Remy made getting to the gym a daily goal. She had always been a busy stay-at-home mom, but now faced with this newfound time, she decided to use it productively.

"I work out for 2½ hours a day, every day (except Sunday), and I am still 50 pounds overweight!" she told me. "This makes no sense at all. I watch all my friends in my exercise classes or on the elliptical next to me, and they seem to be getting in better shape. My weight has not budged since I started working out a year ago. In fact, I am the biggest I have ever been in my life!"

Obviously, there was something amiss. We went over her 3-day diet recall. A typical day would be to grab a granola bar before the gym, go out to lunch after the gym with friends, run errands, come home, and make sure dinner was ready for her husband and son. At lunch, a ravenous Remy (a 2 on the HD scale) would be excited for her meal because she had put in a good workout that day and only had a granola bar so far. She would always try to make good decisions like ordering a salad, but it was often loaded with nuts, dried cranberries, cheese, and a yummy dressing, of course. A piece of bread would usually get snuck in there as well. "What's the big deal?" she would say to herself. "I work out."

Then she'd be full (an 8 on the Hunger Determination Scale) and busy. Many times she wouldn't eat again until around 7:00 p.m. with her son and husband. Dinner would consist of a protein, like steak or chicken, and a starch, most likely pasta (her son was on the football team, so this was a staple). Trying to be good, she would fill her plate with tons of protein (at this point she would be a 2 on the scale), but the pasta would make an appearance on her plate. (After all, she works out!) Remy's biggest question to me was, "Why am I a gym rat and still fat?"

Here are the typical Chubby Perpetual Exerciser health derailers.

- **Skewed workout reporting.** Breaking down Remy's workouts, we discovered she was not actually working out for 2½ hours! Accounting for time spent traveling around the gym, talking to fellow gym rats, and answering some texts, we concluded Remy was working out solidly for 60 minutes (some days with more effort than others). An hour is great, but realistically you are burning 500 calories at most (that's a kick-butt workout with full effort). The cheese and nuts on the salad can easily take care of that.

- **No preparation and planning.** Not planning out your morning breakfast and not being equipped with snacks for all those hours between lunch and dinner is going to lead to big trouble. Eating a sugary, processed snack before the gym does not HD satiate. It is better to have planned food choices before the gym so you can work out more efficiently.
- **Using gym-going as a license to eat whatever.** This is self-explanatory!
- **Overindulging in protein.** Just because there are no carbs in animal protein does not make it limitless. It still has calories and fat! People who exercise a lot are commonly under this false assumption.

The Plump Know-It-All

When Vivienne—an attractive, recently married twentysomething with a high-powered job—first walked into my office, she made sure to let me know she was no stranger to dieting and restricting calories. (She is, what I call, a typical "fad-diet junkie.") "I know what to do," she told me. "I lost 20 pounds before my wedding, but I have gained half of it back and am fed up because my old tricks are not working."

Vivienne's 3-day diet recall revealed that she would start her day off with an English muffin and some I Can't Believe It's Not Butter! spray (it's only 100 calories). To get through her busy work morning, she would have two large iced coffees with low-fat milk and packets of Sweet'N Low to give her energy. Lunch would always be the "perfect" salad, with lettuce, cucumbers, tomatoes, avocados, and olive oil and lemon. Then she'd have more coffee. After work she would go home to have the perfect no-carb dinner with her husband. And she would always end the night with a diet ice cream bar. ("Come on it's 100 calories so it's no big deal!" she told me.) Her recall also revealed that she would binge on chips or sugar cereals around three times a week. ("It's stressful to be so perfect all of the time!" she exclaimed.)

Typical Plump Know-It-All health derailers include:

- **Filling up on artificially sweetened foods.** Often I find that clients fill up on these foods because they are free of or low in calories. But this actually hinders weight loss and is a habit that needs to be broken. See the "Artificial Sweeteners" section in Chapter 7 for reasons why.
- **Being a perfectionist by day and a pig by night.** When you are always restricting food and are hungry, it is not surprising to have a binge

breakdown, which for many people happens at night when they are "relaxing."

- **Making wrong "right" decisions.** There are better decisions that can be made to accomplish HD satiation, even when it comes to the "perfect" salad.

The Busy Mama

Maya walked into my office in the evening, out of breath, messy hair pulled back. Her energy made me nervous; I wanted to tell her to take a deep breath and relax. Maya, a school guidance counselor with three children, started her days at 5:45 a.m. and ended them at 10:00 p.m. "I just don't know how to get a handle on my diet," she said, close to tears. "I just have no time to even think about it, and I have no idea what to do." She wanted to be a healthy mom, a happier wife, and more present at her job.

Maya's 3-day diet recall revealed that in the morning, she was way too busy to think about breakfast. She would always get a coffee on her way to work, and on a good day she would have an energy bar before walking into her office. She'd try to not graze on the cookies and cakes put out for staff members, but sometimes she would be too weak to resist. She'd bring lunch because she wanted to be good. Typically, it'd be a sandwich consisting of wheat bread, turkey, and cheese, which she would make while preparing her children's lunches. When she got home at 3:30 p.m. to greet her kids, she would be starving and munch on all their after-school snacks along with them. After shuttling her children to dance class, basketball, and gymnastics, she would typically pick up dinner from a pizza place or deli. At night she'd binge on high-carb snacks while watching her favorite TV shows. (This was her time to unwind, and she looked forward to peace, quiet, and her comfort foods.)

Busy Mama health derailers are:

- **Skipping meals.** Not having breakfast in the morning is a habit that needs to be broken. It slows down your metabolism. In Maya's case, it was also leading to bad food decisions at work.
- **Choosing highly processed, high-carb energy bars.** These bars are not the best HD decision to replace a meal.
- **Not properly building meals.** It's wonderful that Maya took the time to make her own lunch. However, on the HD plan you will learn to

build meals that will have you feeling like a 7 on the HD Scale afterward and feel satiated for several hours. A sandwich with turkey and cheese is not the best choice.

- **Eating "just to eat."** Eating in front of the TV can lead to mindless overindulgence.
- **Not preparing snacks.** The afternoon is long, so it is important to always prepare the right snacks that keep you from falling to a 2 or 3 on the Hunger Determination Scale.

The Constant Socializer

When Stan walked through my door, I liked him right off the bat. The owner of a successful auto parts business, Stan was in his midfifties with a personality larger than life. "I love to live my life to the fullest," Stan said to me with a smile. "I have worked hard, and now it's time to enjoy my friends and family. The problem is, I have gotten so heavy that I am concerned about my health. I want to be healthy and enjoy the fruits of my labors."

Stan's 3-day diet recall told a lot about why he was overweight. Namely, he was *always* eating at restaurants—no exaggeration. He would have breakfast meetings at diners, extravagant take-out lunches in the office with clients, and decadent dinners out most nights of the week. And he would have at least one or two drinks four nights a week. Stan was always entertaining others and having a ball.

When I pointed out the obvious—that ordering buffalo wings and chicken parmigiana all the time was going to make this a difficult journey—Stan told me he understood what I was saying, but he liked to order "like a man" for his clients and friends. He wanted to take pleasure in his food. Stan was aware of many of the bad habits he had fallen into, and he also knew that changes had to be made. For Stan, this was literally a matter of life and death, and he was ready.

I constantly find that Constant Socializers struggle with these common health derailers.

- **Going out for every meal.** When you are going out this much, you have to understand that you're not the chef in the kitchen and the calories will add up, often without you even knowing where they're hidden. This applies even when you order perfectly, so it obviously applies to ordering decadent meals like Stan does. (There's a reason restaurant mashed potatoes taste richer than your homemade ones: It's because chefs will often add more butter than you ever would, knowing all you'll be aware of is the taste.)

- **Being embarrassed to order "like a girl."** I hear this a lot from men. They somehow feel that if they order light and healthy, they'll be judged by the guys or even their date. To all the men out there: I have a feeling your loved ones would rather you order healthfully and live long than watch you clog up your arteries and expand your waistline.
- **Drinking alcohol several times a week.** This can tack on the calories while lowering your eating inhibitions. Plus, all calories are not created equal. I'll talk about this in Chapter 7.

The Enormous Iron Man

Evan was referred to me by a personal trainer friend of mine. He was training for an Ironman triathlon, so I was expecting a fairly in-shape guy who just needed some sports nutrition advice to walk into my office. I was well aware of the rigorous training schedule that my friend was putting him through each day. Contrary to the gym rat, who isn't always working at full capacity, Evan was part of a training group that went through a steady, challenging workout 6 out of 7 days a week. So when he walked in the door, I was taken aback. Evan—who was in his late thirties with a demanding job and two young children—was at least 40 pounds overweight. He explained to me that he really wanted to understand why the pounds weren't flying off. He was so dedicated to the program, and part of the reason he decided to participate in the Ironman competition was to get into shape. "I have never been so committed to a fitness program in my life, and there is nothing happening to my weight," he said to me. "In fact, my body is slowing me down. I am just staying the same, and I am so confused."

Evan's 3-day diet recall exposed numerous bad habits that he was oblivious of. He would always start his workout early in the morning. Before he met with his trainer, he would have an energy drink, and after his rigorous workout, he would have a 300-calorie protein drink (we figured this out). Starving from his tough workout, he would order an egg sandwich with cheese and home fries once he got to work. And his daily eating habits were a disaster from there. Evan was completely mindless of all the things he put into his body. He ate whatever he felt like.

In addition, he would consume protein bars (at 400 calories a bar!), drinks, and shakes like they were going out of style. He believed that it was helping him build up more muscle. There was one story he told me about going to a Yankees game with his son. He hadn't eaten since lunch and was starving, so he ate one of his bars (second of the day) on the way, and when he got to the game he ordered a cheesesteak sandwich, a beer, and a pretzel to have the "ballgame experience." The calories from this episode alone added up to 2,200. And this was at the end of his day. Really, most days he was consuming 4,000 to 5,000 calories! He was floored by this revelation. He was just totally unaware of the bad decisions he was making, and after his recall, it was no mystery as to why his training hadn't translated to pounds lost.

Here are the Enormous Iron Man health derailers.

- **Consuming too many supplemental protein bars, shakes, and drinks.** Meal replacement products are big business, and many people who start to work out (especially men) stock up on these items and use them as snacks. The fact is, many of these calorie-dense bars and drinks are high in carbs, use artificial sweeteners or sugar, contain synthetic protein, and have no fiber. They do not keep you full for very long either.
- **Mindless eating all day long.** Devouring high-calorie shakes and bars counts as eating! If you are not conscientious about your meals as well, the calories can add up so fast that any hard work to get your body in shape is just canceled out. Always be mindful of what you put in your body.
- **Never being prepared with meals/snacks during the day, especially considering a vigorous workout, work, and family schedule.** This is most likely the reason for making "bad" choices while out and about. Anticipating how hungry you'll be at certain parts of the day will help you make an eating plan.

While some of the health derailers experienced by the diet characters I just talked about might be familiar to you as diet no-nos (like skipping breakfast), others can be insidious, like letting 6 hours go by in the afternoon without a thought of food or always grabbing seconds without thinking. Before embarking on the HD food plan, think about your own derailers. Did you relate to any of these characters? This is a good time to take your own 3-day diet recall to help uncover events and habits that might be sabotaging your weight-loss efforts. It will also reveal your typical eating patterns, which is very important on the HD plan. You will learn to build your snacks and meals the HD way in the following chapters, but the first step on this journey is understanding your "script."

The Hunger Determination Scale is a valuable tool as well because recording your hunger data gives you insight into why you may be falling into many of these bad habits. Use the scale and the food log sheets (on page 240 or at decisionnutrition.com) to expose your derailers. The logs

CAN YOU SAY YES TO ANY OF THE FOLLOWING HEALTH DERAILERS?

- ☐ You consistently run out the door in the morning without eating.
- ☐ You are always too busy in the middle of the day to eat lunch.
- ☐ You start your day proud and restrictive and then fall apart at the seams later in the day with a carton of ice cream.
- ☐ You look at the time and realize you haven't eaten in, like, 7 hours.
- ☐ You are ravenous at lunchtime. You will eat anything that's in your path.
- ☐ You are on edge by dinnertime. No one wants to get in your way until you ingest something.
- ☐ You raid the cabinets every afternoon like a beast.
- ☐ You pick at your children's/spouse's/friends' meals or snacks because you think that will make the calories not count.
- ☐ You eat in front of the TV or computer and then realize you have eaten an entire bag of chips.
- ☐ You use exercise as the reason you can eat whatever and whenever you want.
- ☐ You eat foods with unrecognizable ingredients.
- ☐ You only eat foods that will taste the same if you ate them a year from now. (No fresh foods!)
- ☐ You constantly eat meal-replacement bars/shakes as snacks or meals.
- ☐ You use coffee as a between-meals filler. (Up to two cups of coffee a day is okay, but not as a food replacement!)
- ☐ You reward yourself at night with a sleeve of Oreos.
- ☐ You eat everything in sight at night because you are still hungry and can't sleep.

will also be used throughout the HD plan to keep track of your food intake and your new HD eating patterns.

See the section below for a list of many of the health derailers I have seen in my practice (and participated in myself!). We all can relate to at least one of these derailers (if not more). You need to be aware of your own bad habits and then make the decision to address them. Please check off any of the health derailers you relate to. Once you do this, your HD journey is under way.

So we've covered your current habits and possible self-defeating storylines! *Are you ready to rewrite your script?*

- ☐ You never eat anything green.
- ☐ You overeat protein foods (like chicken, steak, and turkey) because they are carbohydrate free.
- ☐ You never have a plan for any of your meals or snacks.
- ☐ You find yourself thinking about food during your busy day but push the thought aside because you have no time or appetizing options around.
- ☐ You overload on foods with empty carbohydrates, like chips, pastas, and breads.
- ☐ You have a buffet of take-out menus and use them a lot.
- ☐ You don't remember the last time you ate a meal at home.
- ☐ You are embarrassed to order healthy at a restaurant because you will sound high-maintenance.
- ☐ You drink alcohol more than twice a week.
- ☐ You use artificial sweetener packets like crazy.
- ☐ You weigh yourself three times a day.
- ☐ You never weigh yourself. You don't even own a scale. (There will be a section on this in the next chapter.)
- ☐ You eat heart-healthy foods—like olive oil, avocados, and nuts—like they are free of calories. (These foods still count!)
- ☐ Your portions look like they could feed a linebacker.
- ☐ You give up on a healthy eating plan if you don't see massive results immediately.
- ☐ You rely on ready-made foods (from a service or market) or frozen entrées for most meals.
- ☐ You compare your body type to your mother's, your friend's, your spouse's, a celebrity's.

PAUL, 50,
Lost 22 Pounds

Before HD: One day I looked in the mirror and I took a picture of myself. I didn't like what I saw. It was my "fat picture." And I decided I didn't want to look like that anymore.

Initial goal: At the time, I was in the process of training for a marathon. I had been a workout person for a number of years. And despite all the exercise I did, I wasn't losing any weight. So I was in good physical shape but still heavy. I wanted to figure out how to change that.

Starting strong: It's really easy to just eat whatever's in front of you, that piece of pizza or hamburger. On the HD plan you actually have to think about what you're eating.

New foods: Eating chia seeds and oatmeal is a great part of my day. All the green vegetables and salads and the Good Decisions Soup are delicious.

Lesson learned: Shopping for your own fresh vegetables and then preparing and cooking them (or storing them for later) is not hard to do. It's just not that time consuming. And, as a result, you really start to think about what you're eating.

Inspiring words: I had a Super Bowl party, and I laid out all healthy snacks. And everybody was happy! My friends who came over looking for chips and dip and all the other typical unhealthy stuff instead found baked kale chips and yogurt-oriented dips and other healthy snacks that Keren introduced me to. Nobody complained. People even asked me for recipes.

4

PUT IT IN WRITING—YOUR **HD WORK**

*"Commitment means staying loyal
to what you said you were going to do
long after the mood you said it in has left you."*

—UNKNOWN

Where do you see yourself in 3 months? What about 6 months? A year?

Everyone is different. My client Maya wanted to get back to her pre-baby weight (her "baby" is now 5). You might want to slip yourself into a Herve Leger dress and look fit or walk around the pool comfortably on your next vacation, with no cover-up necessary. Perhaps you just want to be able to run around with your kids on weekends with more energy. This is the fun part—your time to think about all the things you desire from gaining control over your eating and weight. But trust me: Your wish list can become your truth.

I find that it is helpful to write down your desires so that you can see them in black and white. As I have been saying all along, there will be bumps in the road. When you come across a tough decision or a bad week on your HD journey, just take a step back, read your own words, and get back to it.

Do not lose sight of your ultimate goal.

Here are the exact steps I walk my clients through in order to help them achieve success. First, I ask my clients what it is they truly want to achieve. Then they write down what it will feel like when they've attained their goals. I ask them to write affirmatively in the present tense to truly visualize what it feels like to reach their goals. Finally, I have my clients list the decisions they will make to achieve their goals. I encourage them to refer to the health derailers uncovered during the 3-day diet recall and then strategize how they'll overcome them.

Here are some sample responses from my clients.

ON-THE-GO GOBBLER: THERESA

Goal: I want to be able to wear a bathing suit in front of my family (instead of hiding) on the reunion cruise.

How It Will Feel: On the deck of the cruise ship, for all of my fellow passengers—and my whole extended family!—to see, I'm wearing one of those sarongs you tie at the hip instead of my usual caftan. And my ever-critical cousin Rachel actually compliments me on how thin my waist is.

Decisions: (1) I'll start to make and bring healthy lunches to work instead of eating whatever my coworkers order. (2) I'll stock up on healthy snacks so I don't overindulge at dinner. (3) I'll stop drinking my two glasses of wine while I'm unwinding from my workday and watching *The Bachelor* and *Keeping Up with the Kardashians.*

THE BUSY MAMA: MAYA

Goal: I want to fit into my 5-year-old prepregnancy jeans again!

How It Will Feel: My old jeans slip on easily, and they zip up without a hitch. But they're so out of style that I have to go shopping for new ones—and a few other items besides!

Decisions: (1) I'll stop finishing everything on my daughter's plate. (2) I'll resist having cake and ice cream at every kid's birthday party. (3) I will no longer mindlessly eat in front of the TV.

THE ENORMOUS IRON MAN: EVAN

Goal: I want to lose my beer belly by the time I compete in the Ironman competition so I can improve my finish time.

How It Will Feel: I am sleek and swimming faster than ever before, slicing through the water without feeling the drag of excess weight on my belly. When I'm running, my knees no longer feel the impact of the 40 extra pounds I was carrying; they are thankful that they might not need to be replaced in 10 years after all!

Decisions: (1) I'll take a fruit and a healthy protein with me as a snack to eat before my morning workout so I am not so ravenous, and I'll focus on a healthier breakfast afterward instead of grabbing my usual fast-food egg sandwich. (2) I will be more mindful of my consumption of high-calorie protein shakes and bars. (3) I'll limit my protein portions to 6 ounces, not 16, like I've been eating!

Now it's your turn. Go to page 238 or decisionnutrition.com for a blank HD contract that you can start to fill out for yourself. Are you ready to make the decision to live your life in HD? Can you commit to the plan? Please do not underestimate the power of your decisions and your affirmations to yourself. Your written words, your spoken words, and the messages you tell yourself can help you get where you want to be with your health and body.

While I am my clients' advocate, I only see each of them once a week. Like all of them, you will be in control of your thoughts every day, and they do make a difference. This contract will serve as a reminder of your ultimate goal and the changes that only you can affect with your daily decisions. You'll track your weight weekly, but remember that weight loss isn't always a linear progression and your goal is more than a number on the scale. This contract will serve as a reminder of why you are undertaking this journey.

THE IMPORTANCE OF FOOD LOGGING

I know this is a sore subject for so many people who embark on a new eating lifestyle. We have so many things on our to-do lists already that adding one more task seems overwhelming. I understand. I am going to level with you, though. In my practice, the clients who have succeeded (not all, but most) have been very efficient at keeping track of their daily food intake and hunger data. Now, some clients never food log and still thrive. The problem is, say you don't log and there's a week where the scale goes up, to your surprise. Since you have no record of what you ate and drank over that week, it's harder to figure out how certain foods affect you. Think about it. Can you even remember what you ate yesterday? You almost certainly don't remember what you had for lunch 4 days ago.

On the other hand, say you have an amazing week. Then it's wonderful to look back at the meals and snacks that you ate while *losing* weight. It's all very valuable information. In addition, accountability is very important. If you are meeting a trainer at the gym at 6:00 a.m., you will (as hard as it is) most likely drag your butt there. Why? You made a commitment to a person who is counting on you to show up.

So I want you to make this commitment to *yourself* and keep track of what you put in your body for 12 weeks on the HD plan. Show up for yourself. You will discover so much about yourself. I have clients who were consistent loggers and lost 40 pounds. I still see them for check-ins, and they are maintaining their new weight and no longer need to keep a food diary. You will get there too. For now, track your food every day using the HD Food Log template on page 240. Yes, it may seem annoying (at first). But it is important to do for 12 weeks. It's your HD work.

ON-THE-GO GOBBLER: THERESA

A page from Theresa's diet recall revealed why her scale was not budging. As you look over a typical beginning to her workweek, see if her health derailers are apparent to you. Be sure to look at her Hunger Determination (HD) Scale recordings, which reveal why she is making many of her present decisions. The HD Scale number represents readings before and after meals. The modifications in the HD Decisions column are suggestions for Theresa to ***Start Strong***. (See page 66 for the Starting Strong guidelines.)

MONDAY

MEAL: *Breakfast* **LOCATION:** *Deli* **TIME:** *7:00 a.m.* **HD SCALE:** *5/6*

DECISIONS	HEALTH DERAILERS	HD IMPROVEMENTS
1 whole wheat scooped-out bagel 2 scrambled eggs 1 piece Muenster cheese 1 coffee with skim milk	Lacking high-hydro food Portion of eggs and bagel need modification Cheese is an IF Caution: Restaurant prep is usually with more oil or butter	Warm lemon water before coffee; almond milk in coffee ½ scooped-out bagel, or better yet be prepared with an HD-friendly carbohydrate like a Decision Nutrition Chia Bagel 5 egg whites or 1 egg and 2 egg whites Add high-hydro vegetables like onions, red peppers, and spinach No cheese Watch butter or oil

MEAL: *AM Snack* **TIME:** *11:00 a.m.* **HD SCALE:** *3/2*

DECISIONS	HEALTH DERAILERS	HD IMPROVEMENTS
None	Not prepared with a snack at work for long morning stretch Ignoring uncomfortable hunger	Always be prepared with a snack 6 ounces Fage plain Greek yogurt 1 cup berries 1 tablespoon hydro-boosting chia seeds for long morning stretch to lunch in order to stay HD satiated Water

MEAL: *Lunch* **LOCATION:** *Takeout* **TIME:** *2:30 p.m.* **HD SCALE:** *1/9*

DECISIONS	HEALTH DERAILERS	HD IMPROVEMENTS
Caesar Salad (3 cups romaine lettuce, ¼ cup Caesar creamy dressing, ½ cup Parmesan cheese, and ½ cup croutons) Two 4-ounce chicken breasts 1 roll 3 small chocolate chip cookies 1 Diet Coke	7 hours since last meal! HD Scale before a meal should be no less than 4 and after, no more than 7 Should not have carb at this meal; high-hydro carb saved for later No high-hydro vegetables in salad Hunger led to overportions and bad decisions and foods from IF list	Salad including six high-hydro vegetables (See Creating the Ultimate HD Salad, page 161) Eliminate heavy dressing and use balsamic or red wine vinegar instead Eliminate one chicken breast Eliminate roll and cookies Seltzer with lemon

MEAL: *PM Snack* **TIME:** *5:00 p.m.* **HD SCALE:** *7/6*

DECISIONS	HEALTH DERAILERS	HD IMPROVEMENTS
None	Still full from lunch	1 apple 2 tablespoons chia peanut butter Water

MEAL: *Dinner* **LOCATION:** *Chinese Restaurant* **TIME:** *8:30 p.m.* **HD SCALE:** *2/8*

DECISIONS	HEALTH DERAILERS	HD IMPROVEMENTS
2 handfuls of Chinese crunchy noodles 10 shrimp with 2 cups mixed vegetables (broccoli, snow peas, cabbage, and zucchini) 1 cup white rice Diet Coke 1 glass of pinot grigio	Once again HD scale has dipped below a 4 before dinner and above a 7 after Hunger led to bad food decisions Overportioned meal Artificial sweetener drink (IF) Wine on IF list	High-hydro vegetables present, which is great, but prepared in high-sodium and oil sauce. Order steamed. 7 shrimp 2 cups of vegetables is fine, if steamed Switch out white rice for brown rice and decrease to ½ cup (¼ of your plate) Seltzer with lemon No wine

MEAL: *Nighttime Snack* **TIME:** *11:00 p.m.* **HD SCALE:** *7/8*

DECISIONS	HEALTH DERAILERS	HD IMPROVEMENTS
4 handfuls of granola	Not hungry Entire day was carb and sugar loaded, which led to this bad decision	Should just go to bed! If using HD plan and want a sweet, eat any high-hydro fruit.

CHUBBY PERPETUAL EXERCISER: REMY

A page from Remy's diet recall reveals why she spends so much time at the gym with no results. See if you can spot her health derailers materialize as she goes through a very typical Tuesday.

TUESDAY

MEAL: *Breakfast* **TIME:** *8:00 a.m.* **HD SCALE:** *4/4*

DECISIONS	HEALTH DERAILERS	HD IMPROVEMENTS
Special K Protein Bar Coffee with half-and-half	Unwrapping food for breakfast is an HD no-no. Bar is not satiating. Scale number remained the same, and she is about to go to the gym. Lacking high-hydro foods	Warm lemon water ½ cup rolled oats 1 cup strawberries 1 tablespoon chia seeds (hydro-boost before gym) Coffee with unsweetened almond milk

MEAL: *AM Snack* **TIME:** *Noon* **HD SCALE:** *2/3*

DECISIONS	HEALTH DERAILERS	HD IMPROVEMENTS
Banana	Banana is an HD-friendly fruit avoided in Start Strong Should be prepared with appropriate HD snack since not meeting a friend for lunch until 1:15 p.m.	1 apple

MEAL: *Lunch* **LOCATION:** *Restaurant* **TIME:** *1:15 p.m.* **HD SCALE:** *2/8*

DECISIONS	HEALTH DERAILERS	HD IMPROVEMENTS
3 breadsticks Kale salad with tomatoes, cucumber, beets, asparagus, ½ avocado, and 10 walnuts 1 ounce goat cheese 8 ounces grilled salmon 4 tablespoons raspberry vinaigrette 2 glasses of water	HD scale demonstrates insufficient high-hydro foods to this point, which led to bread basket attack. Too many MUFAs. Must pick either avocado or walnuts and modify portions Salmon overportioned Too much oil-based dressing	No breadsticks 6 walnuts ***or*** ¼ avocado 4 ounces salmon Nice presence of hydrophilic vegetables but need to watch the dressing portion Reduce to 1 tablespoon of restaurant's dressing or go for unlimited vinegar instead

MEAL: *PM Snack* **TIME:** *3:45 p.m.* **HD SCALE:** *4/5*

DECISIONS	HEALTH DERAILERS	HD IMPROVEMENTS
½ cup plain pasta while preparing dinner	Mindless eating of pasta. It still counts!	Have a mindful HD snack with high-hydro foods so not uncomfortably hungry before dinner. High-hydro vegetables like peppers, sugar snap peas, and carrots 4 ounces hummus 1 tablespoon chia seeds

MEAL: *Dinner* **LOCATION:** *Restaurant* **TIME:** *8:30 p.m.* **HD SCALE:** *2/8*

DECISIONS	HEALTH DERAILERS	HD IMPROVEMENTS
One 5-ounce breaded cutlet 1½ cups pasta ¾ cup marinara sauce 1 cup mushrooms 2 tablespoons of Parmesan cheese Crystal Light	Too many carbs with breaded cutlet and pasta (including above snack) Need to mix mushroom (HD-friendly vegetable) with a high-hydro vegetable for satiation Cheese on IF list Replace pasta with a high-hydro carb like quinoa Artificial flavor drink (IF)	Eliminate breading from chicken and reduce to 4-ounce serving Add asparagus with the mushrooms ½ cup low-sugar pasta sauce No cheese Make quinoa instead of pasta and modify to ½ cup (¼ plate) Seltzer with lemon

MEAL: *Nighttime Snack* **TIME:** *11:00 p.m.* **HD SCALE:** *4/6*

DECISIONS	HEALTH DERAILERS	HD IMPROVEMENTS
Whole container of pineapple (2 cups)	HD-friendly fruit not in Start Strong Portion too big	Poached Cinnamon Pears, page 232, or Free Frozen Fruit Skewer, page 222

PLUMP KNOW-IT-ALL: VIVIENNE

Vivienne's diet recall exposes her dependence on "diet" foods and how her constant restricting makes living in HD a challenge. Here is an example of her Wednesday diet recall. See what her health derailers are:

WEDNESDAY

MEAL: *Breakfast* **TIME:** *7:45 a.m.* **HD SCALE:** *4/5*

DECISIONS	HEALTH DERAILERS	HD IMPROVEMENTS
Water 2 hard-cooked egg whites 1 piece whole wheat toast 1 tablespoon diet strawberry jelly	Lacking high-hydro foods Low-calorie meal Diet jelly is artificial and not nutritious (IF)	Warm water with lemon Replace wheat toast with a high-hydro carb like oatmeal (make Chia-Oat Pancake, page 177) Chia-Raspberry Smash, page 185, in place of jelly

MEAL: *AM Snack* **LOCATION:** *Restaurant* **TIME:** *11:30 a.m.* **HD SCALE:** *3/4*

DECISIONS	HEALTH DERAILERS	HD IMPROVEMENTS
1 super-size large iced coffee light with skim milk and 3 Sweet'N Low Skinny Cow Heavenly Crisp Bar (110 calories)	Lacking high-hydro foods Artificial foods with bar and Sweet'N Low HD scale a 4 after this snack, so not really satiated	Iced coffee light with unsweetened vanilla almond milk 1 stevia packet High-hydro vegetables like peppers, carrots, sugar snap peas Onion Yogurt Dip, page 182

MEAL: *Lunch* **TIME:** *1:00 p.m.* **HD SCALE:** *3/4*

DECISIONS	HEALTH DERAILERS	HD IMPROVEMENTS
2 cups iceberg lettuce 2 tomatoes, chopped 1 whole avocado 4 tablespoons diet ranch dressing Diet Coke	No high-hydro vegetables Too much avocado No protein Artificial ingredients in dressing and soda	2 cups kale 1 cup steamed broccoli 2 tomatoes, cut up Chopped zucchini 1 cup kidney beans Good Decisions Dressings choice (page 189–192) or unlimited vinegar Seltzer with lemon

MEAL: *PM Snack* **TIME:** *4:30 p.m.* **HD SCALE:** *3/4*

DECISIONS	HEALTH DERAILERS	HD IMPROVEMENTS
Super-size iced coffee light with skim milk 3 Sweet'N Low	HD scale indicates still hungry Using coffee as way to divert hunger Not eating until 7:00 p.m. so needs to be prepared with an HD snack More artificial ingredients	Skip coffee 1 apple 15 almonds

MEAL: *Dinner* **TIME:** *7:00 p.m.* **HD SCALE:** *2/6*

DECISIONS	HEALTH DERAILERS	HD IMPROVEMENTS
Two 6-ounce turkey burgers from butcher 1 cup broccoli sautéed in 4 tablespoons olive oil 2 Diet Cokes	HD scale before too low and still indicates not full after Too much protein Too much olive oil No high-hydro carbohydrate Artificial drinks	1 cup Good Decisions Soup, page 195 One 4-ounce turkey burger ½ cup brown rice 2 cups broccoli sautéed HD way (page 166) Seltzer with lemon Add more high-hydro vegetables

MEAL: *Nighttime Snack* **TIME:** *10:30 p.m.* **HD SCALE:** *2/8*

DECISIONS	HEALTH DERAILERS	HD IMPROVEMENTS
8 ounces Baked Lays Potato Chips (almost whole bag) Skinny Cow Ice Cream Bar Diet Coke	"Diet" day caught up, and she crashed binging on potato chips and ice cream (the lighter versions, of course) Huge jump in HD scale at bedtime Too many carbs and artificial ingredients Artificial drink	1 cup raspberries with HD freebie like Vanilla Agar Pudding, page 220

BUSY MAMA: MAYA

Take a look at a typical busy Thursday for Maya. Is it easy to see the health derailers that emerge and inhibit her from living in HD?

THURSDAY

MEAL: *Breakfast* **TIME:** *7:30 p.m.* **HD SCALE:** *3/3*

DECISIONS	HEALTH DERAILERS	HD IMPROVEMENTS
Coffee with ¼ cup half-and-half	Skipping breakfast before a busy work morning ahead	1 packet instant plain oatmeal 1 cup raspberries 1 tablespoon chia seeds (hydro-booster) Add breakfast with high-hydro foods to avoid HD scale dip later on

MEAL: *AM Snack* **TIME:** *10:30 p.m.* **HD SCALE:** *1/3*

DECISIONS	HEALTH DERAILERS	HD IMPROVEMENTS
10 Hershey Kisses from bowl display at work	Bad decision made because skipped breakfast. High-calorie IF and not even satiated after (HD scale = 3) Not prepared with HD snack	1 orange 24 pistachios

MEAL: *Lunch* **TIME:** *Noon* **HD SCALE:** *3/6*

DECISIONS	HEALTH DERAILERS	HD IMPROVEMENTS
2 pieces of white bread 5 ounces turkey breast 1 slice American cheese 3 tablespoons honey-mustard dressing 1-ounce bag pretzels Water	Lacking high-hydro foods Overportioned turkey Too many carbs Honey-mustard high in sugar Cheese is an IF	Start with Broccoli Soup, page 193 Replace white bread with HD-friendly carb option like a La Tortilla wrap 4 ounces turkey Add high-hydro vegetables like julienned carrots, zucchini, and cabbage Replace honey-mustard with Dijon mustard No pretzels

MEAL: *PM Snack* **TIME:** *4:00 p.m.* **HD SCALE:** *2/6*

DECISIONS	HEALTH DERAILERS	HD IMPROVEMENTS
1 Nutrigrain bar ½ cup Goldfish snack crackers	HD scale dip leads to poor, nonnutritious food decisions Not prepared with HD snacks	Chia Cacao Yogurt, page 219

MEAL: *Dinner* **LOCATION:** *Italian Takeout* **TIME:** *8:00 p.m.* **HD SCALE:** *2/8*

DECISIONS	HEALTH DERAILERS	HD IMPROVEMENTS
2 cups eggplant Parmesan 1 cup spaghetti	Lack of high-hydro foods Dish overloaded with cheese, carbs, and oil No protein Always taking out, so need to make better decisions Needs to start planning meals at home more	4 ounces grilled chicken Already used allotted carbs for day 2 cups steamed spinach with a squeeze of lemon Easy prep dinner: Spaghetti squash topped with HD Ratatouille (page 200) and 4 ounces chicken

MEAL: *Nighttime Snack* **TIME:** *11:30 p.m.* **HD SCALE:** *7/8*

DECISIONS	HEALTH DERAILERS	HD IMPROVEMENTS
3 cups tortilla chips with salsa	Eating when not hungry (HD scale = 7) So many empty carbs in her day	1 cup baked kale chips with ¼ cup salsa

THE CONSTANT SOCIALIZER: STAN

Stan's very social lifestyle remained throughout his HD journey. He did, however, make radical changes to what he was eating and to his eating patterns. Here is a page from his Start Strong food log. There are no changes needed! He was living in HD, losing weight, and still going out a lot!

FRIDAY

MEAL: *Breakfast* **TIME:** *8:30 a.m.* **HD SCALE:** *3/7*

DECISIONS	HEALTH DERAILERS	HD IMPROVEMENTS
Quick Chia Oatmeal, page 173 1 cup blueberries Coffee with almond milk	None	Made a commitment to have high-hydro meal with chia seeds at home since always out for lunch and dinner HD satiated

MEAL: *AM Snack* **TIME:** *11:30 a.m.* **HD SCALE:** *4/5*

DECISIONS	HEALTH DERAILERS	HD IMPROVEMENTS
1 apple 1 tablespoon almond butter	None	Always prepared in office with HD snacks Feeling fine

MEAL: *Lunch* **LOCATION:** *Business Lunch* **TIME:** *1:00 p.m.* **HD SCALE:** *4/7*

DECISIONS	HEALTH DERAILERS	HD IMPROVEMENTS
Vegetable soup 6 ounces filet of sole Side of steamed string beans and asparagus Water with lemon	None	Good start with soup High-hydro vegetables present HD-friendly protein is the correct portion

MEAL: *Dinner* **LOCATION:** *Japanese restaurant* **TIME:** *7:30 p.m.* **HD SCALE:** *4/7*

DECISIONS	HEALTH DERAILERS	HD IMPROVEMENTS
Miso soup Seaweed salad 1 tuna roll with brown rice 8 pieces salmon sashimi Steamed broccoli	None	Good start with soup Seaweed salad filling and hydrophilic 1 roll = ½ cup brown rice Added sashimi for protein Hydrophylic broccoli—added to satiation

MEAL: *Nighttime Snack* **TIME:** *9:30 p.m.* **HD SCALE:** *4/5*

DECISIONS	HEALTH DERAILERS	HD IMPROVEMENTS
Good Decisions Vanilla Chai Pudding (page 221)	None	Approved HD freebie with hydro-booster to satiate before bed!

TRACKING WEEK-TO-WEEK WEIGHT RESULTS

I love the HD contract as a source of inspiration. It is so very important to remember why you picked up this book in the first place and what living in HD means to you. Let me stress once again that what you envision for yourself on day 1 does not happen on day 2, day 10, or even day 20. It's a long process. Therefore I find it very helpful to show my clients other HD plan participants' week-to-week weight results so they can see how a 12-week journey unfolds differently for every person.

While my clients may lose more or less, as a general rule, 20 pounds is a successful weight loss for the 12-week period. I tell clients when they first sit down with me that they can be 20 pounds lighter in 3 months if they make the appropriate changes and stay accountable. Yet, sometime during the 12 weeks, many people get frustrated because they want to lose faster, or they get extremely discouraged by temporary setbacks.

So to encourage those who might be setting unreasonable—or unhealthy—expectations for themselves, the following sample weight-tracking reports portray the real-life 12-week weight-loss journeys of three different clients.

As you can see, weekly weight-loss averages were not 5 or even 2 pounds. There were weeks where 2, 3, and 5 pounds were lost, but on average, successful outcomes were often 1.5 to 1.9 pounds per week.

It's okay to have an up week or a "stuck" week. You are not a robot; you are a human being! You are living life. You don't have the luxury of being in a controlled environment, such as a weight-loss ranch. As I mentioned earlier, for most people weight loss is not a linear progression, and even my most successful clients don't drop weight every week. Please remember this on your journey to your ultimate HD goal.

I stick with my clients to cheer them on and keep them on course when

On-the-Go Gobbler

FEMALE, 5 FEET 5 INCHES TALL, 42 YEARS OLD

START WEIGHT: **176.8 pounds**

GOAL: **130 pounds**

AFTER 12 WEEKS (ROUND 1):
151.2 pounds

AFTER 12 WEEKS (ROUND 2):
139.2 pounds

25.6 pounds lost
(55% of goal) on Round 1
12 pounds lost
(80% of goal) on Round 2

Average weekly weight loss:
1.57 pounds

WEEK	WEIGHT (LBS)	LOSS (LBS)
1	176.80	——
2	170.60	6.20
3	168.00	2.60
4	168.20	+0.20
5	164.00	4.20
6	161.20	2.80
7	159.00	2.20
8	157.40	1.60
9	155.40	2.00
10	153.60	1.80
11	153.00	0.60
12	151.20	1.80
1	149.60	1.60
2	149.00	0.60
3	149.20	+0.20
4	145.60	3.60
5	144.60	1.00
6	146.60	+2.00
7	142.40	4.20
8	141.60	0.80
9	140.60	1.00
10	141.40	+0.80
11	140.00	1.40
12	139.20	0.80

The Busy Mama

FEMALE, 5 FEET 2 INCHES TALL, 37 YEARS OLD

START WEIGHT: **147.2 pounds**

GOAL: **120 pounds**

AFTER 12 WEEKS: **124.8 pounds**

22.4 pounds lost
(82% of goal at end of 12 weeks)

Average weekly weight loss:
1.87 pounds

WEEK	WEIGHT (LBS)	LOSS (LBS)
1	147.20	—
2	142.00	5.20
3	142.40	+0.40
4	139.60	2.80
5	136.00	3.60
6	136.00	—
7	133.40	2.60
8	131.00	2.40
9	131.60	+0.60
10	130.40	1.20
11	130.60	+0.20
12	124.80	5.80

they see their weight go up 0.2, 0.5, 1 pound, or more after working really hard or, on the contrary, after being "bad" the previous week. But because I can't do that via this book, I hope the sample weight-tracking reports help you maintain realistic expectations for your HD journey.

One last point regarding staying sane and being accountable: Pick a day of the week to weigh yourself, and don't weigh yourself at any other times. I suggest Monday or Tuesday morning so you can regroup after weekends, which tend to be less steady both routine- and diet-wise than weekdays for most people. It is also a good idea to stick to the same time of day and use the same scale.

Go to Chapter 6 for detailed week-by-week discussions between Maya and me during her HD journey.

The Enormous Iron Man

MALE, 6 FEET TALL, 39 YEARS OLD

START WEIGHT: **226 pounds**

GOAL: **190 pounds**

AFTER 12 WEEKS: **204.8 pounds**

21.20 pounds lost
(59% of goal at end of 12 weeks)

Average weekly weight loss:
1.77 pounds

WEEK	WEIGHT (LBS)	LOSS (LBS)
1	226.00	—
2	222.80	3.20
3	220.40	2.40
4	219.00	1.40
5	216.60	2.40
6	217.60	+1.00
7	214.40	3.20
8	213.00	1.40
9	212.60	0.40
10	210.20	2.40
11	207.40	2.80
12	204.80	2.60

Why do I recommend you weigh yourself just once a week? I have had clients who weigh themselves three times a day, but weight can fluctuate from day to day, hour to hour. Sometimes they see the number go up and get discouraged when there's really no reason to worry. And if their weight goes down, they can get cocky and not be so quick to pass up the muffins in the office. Stepping on the scale too often generally prompts people to overreact and overcorrect while losing sight of the big picture.

You can record your weekly weight on the weight-tracking log on decisionnutrition.com. Let the log be your guide to how your body is responding to the new HD decisions you are making each week, the progress toward your end weight goal, and your average weekly weight loss.

WEEKLY GOALS

There is a template for weekly goal tracker sheets on page 242 as well as on my Web site, decisionnutrition.com. I consider the weekly goal sheet a short-term contract that you will commit to for the upcoming week. It's just for *one week*, and that's the beauty of it. You have filled out a long-term contract stating where you see yourself at the end of your HD journey, but this weekly goal sheet is about *now* and the week ahead. Clients love them because they leave my office with a sense of direction. The best weekly goals are quick, tactical, memorable, and easy to "win" and reevaluate. There's no guesswork or wiggle room; you either did or didn't accomplish them.

I suggest filling out your weekly goals on the same day you weigh yourself. Remember, these are weekly "promises" you make to yourself, and they can be adjusted according to the upcoming 7 days. For example, if you have two parties for the week, you may commit to being very consistent on the other days of the week and to not going to the parties starving. If you have noticed your weight loss is at a standstill, commit to being more diligent with your food logging that week.

Here, for example, is what Remy the Chubby Perpetual Exerciser's weekly goals might look like.

1. I am going to be very tuned in to my body's signals this week. I will not let 4 hours go by without eating!
2. I will have an appropriate breakfast 1 hour before going to the gym.
3. I will be prepared with a Greek yogurt and a pear for *after* the gym so that when I sit down for lunch I am not ravenous.
4. I will be *much* more aware of my protein portions at each meal.
5. I will log my food intake every day this week.

On the HD plan you make the decisions of what your personal weekly goals will be.

Again, please be realistic about your weekly weight-loss expectations. You are not racing against the clock. I promise that once you practice all the steps on the plan, you will not only lose weight but also learn what really works for your body. You will discover how to live decisively, for life. Remember: Small changes lead to big results!

AMY, 49,
Lost 16 Pounds

Initial goal: I'm 5 feet 3 inches tall, and in terms of sheer numbers, I was small overall. But I didn't want to be one of those middle-aged ladies where you think, "Oh, she must have been cute when she was younger."

Starting strong: I'm a systems person, so give me a plan and I can stick with it. Even though it was hard, having strict rules meant I knew what to do. I also started losing right away, which motivated me to stick with the plan.

New foods: Tofu shirataki noodles.

Never misses: Artificial sweeteners (though I like a diet soda now and then).

Unexpected bonus: My initial reasons for trying the HD plan had to do with how I looked; now I stick to the HD principles because of how I feel.

Lesson learned: Like a lot of people, I thought I was doing things right, and then, through HD, I realized I wasn't as right as I thought I was. For instance, I believed that a Caesar salad for lunch was a healthy choice. There are more calories in there than I thought!

New mantra: Think ahead. If I'm not prepared, I'm going to the vending machine for Twizzlers. Now I keep fruits, 100-calorie packs of almonds, and Greek yogurt in my office.

Sustaining in HD: Change the way you think about food and it becomes second nature. And you can always do it; it's not like you need special stuff or equipment.

Inspiring words: I feel like myself again!

P2

THE 12-WEEK HD PLAN

5

EATING IN HD—THE HD PLAN GUIDELINES AND CORE FOODS

"When you eat in HD, you live in HD."

—KEREN GILBERT

There's no getting around it: To achieve and maintain a healthy weight, you have to *decide* to maintain healthy eating habits. You will find the core eating principles in this section to be very livable for the long term. The HD plan emphasizes high-hydrophilic (high-hydro for short) fruits, vegetables, and legumes, and it allows animal proteins and—unlike many diet plans—approved carbohydrates right from the start. On your HD journey, I want you to keep in mind the Hunger Determination Scale and its principles so you can become aware of how the HD plan meals and snacks satisfy.

More good news: The HD plan *encourages* snacking to help support a healthy metabolism and keep you content between meals. In fact, I insist that you don't go more than 4 hours without eating. Also, use hydro-boosting chia seeds throughout the day so that it's easy to remain a 5, 6, or 7 on the Hunger Determination Scale. The core foods on the HD plan will help you avoid both cravings and energy lulls.

The core foods on this plan are divided into the following categories.

High-hydrophilic foods. These "high-hydro" foods consist of specific vegetables, fruits, grains, and legumes. They provide the most water-loving (soluble) fiber you can find at your local supermarket.

HD-friendly foods. I use the term *HD-friendly* for healthy foods full of necessary nutrients but lacking hydrophilic qualities—like certain whole grains, proteins, fruits, and veggies. These should be eaten in combination with high-hydro foods at meals or at snacktimes for the best results.

Hydro-boosters. Chia seeds aid digestion and are packed with nutrients. Their hydrophilic properties help keep you "philled up"; they leave you "feeling like a 5" (after snacks) and HD satiated or a 7 (after meals) on the Hunger Determination Scale. You'll incorporate chia seeds or Chia Gel (page 158) into your meals or snacks at least two to three times per day.

IFs. Infrequent foods—which I call IFs—are not included in the 2-week Start Strong phase. However, they are introduced slowly in limited amounts in Phases 2 and 3. Yes, you will eventually be able to have your favorites, but you have to relearn how to think about them first. I will help you put these foods in their rightful place in your life so that when you have them, you will be fully mindful of the treat and enjoy every bite.

There's an IF list later in this chapter, and I've dedicated Chapter 7 to sharing why these foods should be infrequent and strategies on how to handle adding them. After 12 weeks, you will really understand what formula works best for your body, and these lessons will be yours forever. When you are at the weight that makes you happiest, you will know how to stay there, sustaining in HD forever.

The plan is split into three phases.

Phase 1: Start Strong

Each day you're allotted the following:

- Unlimited high-hydro/HD-friendly vegetables (but no fewer than 4 high-hydro vegetables in your day)
- Up to 3 high-hydro fruits
- Up to 4 high-hydro/HD-friendly proteins
- Up to 2 high-hydro/HD-friendly carbohydrates (at least 1 high-hydro)
- A hydro-boost meal/snack at least twice
- 1 HD-friendly MUFA

In the Start Strong phase, the stress is on clean eating. If you recall the analogy of learning to play the guitar from Chapter 2, you understand that in the beginning your fingers don't naturally know their place on the strings. In the same way, this phase may present changes to your normal eating routine that will initially feel weird, even uncomfortable.

I'd like you to think of Start Strong as a detoxification. You know those radical detox diets that celebs do all the time, where they drink juice for 7 days straight and lose 10 pounds as a result? Well, that kind of detox is not sustainable. When regular eating is resumed, the scale numbers go right back up. But the reason many people claim to feel so energized on these diets is they have eliminated many foods that wreak havoc on their bodies. In Start Strong, you will do the same. You'll just be incorporating more high-hydrophilic veggies, proteins, and fruits and hydro-boosters in the correct combinations at the right times every day so you don't feel deprived.

Your body will feel the difference immediately if you follow the HD-plan guidelines. Does that mean you won't feel like a glass of wine or dessert if you go out to dinner? Not necessarily. Some people have a hard time staying away from foods on the IF (infrequent foods) list—foods like cheese, red meat, processed sweets, and alcohol. But if you can stay strong for 2 weeks, you're well on your way toward incorporating some of your favorite foods back into your routine, only in smarter ways.

I highly recommend staying in the Start Strong phase for at least 2 weeks. It is important to see how satisfied you can feel on the HD plan and how—amazingly—foods you thought were going to be extremely difficult to incorporate turned out to be easy additions and how foods you imagined never being able to give up were eliminated almost painlessly. In this phase, you see that you have options, you are not hungry, and you feel like you are beginning to live in HD: clear and focused.

How do you know you're ready for Start Strong? Here are some things you might hear yourself saying.

"It's time for me to stop my incessant pigging out."

"It's time for me to make a change because I am miserable."

"Whatever I am doing right now is not working."

"I completely relate to feeling ravenous in the afternoon, so I am going to focus on preparing for Start Strong."

Phase 2: Still Focused in HD

Each day you're allotted the following:

- Unlimited high-hydro/HD-friendly vegetables (but no fewer than 4 high-hydro vegetables in your day)
- Up to 3 high-hydro/HD-friendly fruits (at least 2 high-hydro)
- Up to 4 high-hydro/HD-friendly proteins
- Up to 2 high-hydro/HD-friendly carbohydrates (at least 1 high-hydro)
- Hydro-boost a meal/snack at least twice
- 2 HD-friendly MUFA
- Up to 1 IF serving per week

What happens after the first 2 weeks of Start Strong? *You need to stay focused.* You'll stick with the same principles in the Start Strong phase, but you can begin adding one IF a week. You'll continue in the Still Focused in HD phase for 6 weeks and learn an incredible amount about what you are capable of accomplishing. Still Focused means continuing with your food logs, your weight tracking, and your weekly goals. This way, you can keep a close eye on how an IF food affects your weight, which a lot of my clients find very revealing.

Many clients who are feeling good in Start Strong continue that phase for longer than 2 weeks, especially if their bodies are reacting well. You are in this for 12 weeks total, and these are your decisions to make on your HD journey. A journey does not happen overnight. There will be weeks when staying focused is harder than others. There will be instances where you lose focus entirely and experience a bad week of gaining a pound or two. But Still Focused means you realize those setbacks don't define you. Look over the sample weight-tracking reports in Chapter 4 of others who took the HD journey, and continue your work.

Here are some things you might hear yourself saying while Still Focused in HD.

> "Things are going so well; I want to continue on Start Strong for a little while longer."
>
> "I can't believe I had a frozen yogurt with my kids on Sunday and still lost 2 pounds!"

"I need to have a drink this weekend, but I will stay consistent with everything else I am doing."

Phase 3: Soaring in HD

Each day you're allotted the following:

- ○ Unlimited high-hydro/HD-friendly vegetables (but no fewer than 4 high-hydro vegetables in your day)
- ○ Up to 3 high-hydro/HD-friendly fruits (at least 2 high-hydro)
- ○ Up to 4 high-hydro/HD-friendly proteins
- ○ Up to 3 high-hydro/HD-friendly carbohydrates (at least 2 high-hydro)
- ○ Hydro-boost a meal/snack at least twice
- ○ 1 HD-friendly MUFA
- ○ Up to 2 IFs per week

You are flying now. Although everyone is different, many of my clients are 13, 15, 18 pounds lighter at this point. Once you reach the Soaring in HD phase, you have been at it for 8 weeks. You are feeling more in control and have go-to HD meals and snacks that you have come to love.

Your eating patterns and portions have also changed. This is why you are now ready to add one extra carbohydrate per day and two IFs each week. You can begin to be more liberal with your add-ins once you understand how particular foods—say, a bowl of pasta—really affect you. However, if you want a clean week instead, that's great; just go back to what you were doing during Start Strong.

The HD plan is never a diet in which you feel starved. Truthfully, Soaring in HD reflects the formulas that I believe all people who successfully maintain a healthy weight and attitude for years abide by. I certainly do: Soaring in HD is how I live most every week. It's liberating and empowering. When a vacation comes up and the number on the scale begins to creep in the wrong direction, you now have the tools under your belt to get back to where you want to be—where you feel strongest and happiest.

Here are some things you might hear yourself saying while you are Soaring in HD.

"I feel like the way I approach my food decisions has changed permanently."

"I can't believe I went on vacation and didn't gain an ounce."

"I wasn't ready to be so liberal yet. I still have a ways to go to reach my goal, so I am still going to be mindful of the IFs I incorporate."

The real feat is when you reach your HD contract long-term goals. This is what you are working toward. So depending on your situation, the length of these phases may differ for you. You can stay in Start Strong for well beyond 2 weeks. You may feel you're losing sharpness and clarity toward the end of the Soaring phase and decide you need to go back and do Start Strong again and stay there until you're ready to move on. But it will be easier this time because of all you have learned about yourself thus far.

You will *know* when you are on top of the hill. This is when you are comfortably sustaining in HD. Forever.

HD CORE FOODS BY CATEGORY

Don't worry if these lists are a lot to take in. There will be guidance and menu suggestions later, as well as recipes in Chapter 11. For now, read through and familiarize yourself with the following food lists.

High-Hydro Vegetables
Amount: Unlimited (but no fewer than 4 servings per day)

Some clients walk into my office and announce right away, "Oh, just so you know: I hate all vegetables and I refuse to eat them, but I need to lose 50 pounds. What should I do?"

My answer is . . . LEAVE! Lactose intolerant, gluten free, vegan—I can work around all kinds of preferences, habits, and special diets, but vegetables are the centerpiece of healthy food decisions and the HD plan. So I tell all my veggie-phobic clients that they need to make the decision to expand their palates to include vegetables. It's nonnegotiable in my practice, and I assure them they'll thank me for it later.

The following list includes the high-hydro veggies, and they are unlimited on the HD plan. You can eat them raw, steamed, mashed, roasted, or sautéed the HD way (see Chapter 10 for more on styles of cooking). You can also dress veggies with my Good Decisions Dressing recipes on page 189 or with lemon juice or any other HD-plan unlimited spice or condiment on page 82. Fresh or frozen is best because there is generally a lot of sodium added to canned or jarred vegetables. If canned is your only choice, try to find no-salt-added versions.

- ○ Artichokes
- ○ Asparagus
- ○ Bean sprouts
- ○ Beet greens
- ○ Beets
- ○ Bell peppers (all kinds)
- ○ Bok choy
- ○ Broccoli
- ○ Broccoli rabe
- ○ Broccoli slaw
- ○ Brussels sprouts
- ○ Cabbage (all kinds)
- ○ Carrots
- ○ Collard greens
- ○ Dandelion greens
- ○ Green beans
- ○ Jerusalem artichoke
- ○ Jicama
- ○ Kale
- ○ Kohlrabi
- ○ Mustard greens
- ○ Okra
- ○ Onions
- ○ Radishes
- ○ Snow peas
- ○ Spaghetti squash
- ○ Spinach
- ○ Swiss chard
- ○ Sugar snap peas
- ○ Turnip greens
- ○ Turnips
- ○ Yellow squash
- ○ Zucchini

THE DEAL WITH SQUASH

Every part of a squash can be eaten, including the leaves and tender shoots. But there are just so many varieties of squash—in all different shapes and colors—and it can get really confusing when you are confronted with all those choices at the supermarket.

When it comes to squash, the terms *summer* and *winter* are deceiving. Summer types, like zucchini and yellow squash, are in the market all winter long, while winter varieties, like spaghetti squash, appear in late summer and fall as well as winter.

On the HD plan, zucchini, yellow squash, and spaghetti squash are unlimited. Other winter varieties, like acorn squash and butternut squash, are counted as a high-hydro carb.

HD-Friendly Vegetables
Amount: Unlimited in combination with high-hydro vegetables

While HD-friendly vegetables are low calorie, delicious, and nutritious, they have very little water-soluble fiber and, therefore, have little or no hydrophilic functionality. They won't keep you as full as high-hydro veggies, so when you eat these HD-friendly vegetables on their own, and check in on your hunger an hour later, physiologically you'll likely feel unsatisfied. I've seen this with clients struggling to lose weight who tell me of their "diet" salads of iceberg lettuce, cucumbers, tomatoes, and some sort of protein, like grilled chicken breast. Sure, this is a low-calorie meal, but it will not keep you full for very long. It might even sabotage your dieting efforts.

Therefore, while HD-friendly veggies can be eaten in unlimited quantities on the plan, *they must be combined with equal portions or more of high-hydro vegetables.* If you're going to have eggplant, have it with an equal amount of okra; if you're going to eat cucumber, have it with carrots. The combination ensures you get the proper amount of hydration and fiber. In Chapter 10, I will teach you how to build a delicious HD salad that will keep you feeling full for hours.

Again, fresh or frozen vegetables are best; use no-salt-added jarred or canned veggies in a pinch.

- ○ Arugula
- ○ Bibb lettuce (also known as Boston lettuce)
- ○ Cauliflower
- ○ Celery
- ○ Cucumber
- ○ Eggplant
- ○ Endive
- ○ Fennel
- ○ Hearts of palm
- ○ Iceberg lettuce
- ○ Mesclun
- ○ Mushrooms
- ○ Radicchio
- ○ Romaine lettuce
- ○ Tomatoes
- ○ Water chestnuts
- ○ Watercress

High-Hydro Fruits
Amount: Up to 3 servings per day

Fruits are a big part of the HD lifestyle. Packed with vitamins and minerals, fruits can be incorporated into many meals and snacks to satisfy your cravings for sweetness. Many diets don't allow any fruits or strictly limit them because of the high sugar content, but that's not the case here.

As with the veggies, I divide fruits into two categories: high-hydro and HD-friendly. On the HD plan, you can have up to 3 servings of fruit per day. During Start Strong, all 3 servings must be fruits from the high-hydro list; after those 2 weeks, 1 of the 3 can be an HD-friendly fruit.

You want to eat more high-hydro fruits because your body responds better to their natural sugars. The high fiber and water-absorption properties of high-hydro fruits prevent sharp increases in blood glucose, which helps keep cravings at bay.

In general, fruits make for easy, portable snacks and many (like apples and pears) are delicious when baked.

The following fruits are the most hydrophilic. I've included portion or serving sizes throughout.

- Apple—1 medium
- Apricots—2 small
- Blackberries—1 cup
- Blueberries—1 cup
- Clementines—2 whole
- Cranberries—1 cup
- Figs, fresh—3 medium
- Grapefruit—½ large
- Kiwifruit—1 cup, cubed
- Mango—1 cup, cubed
- Orange—1 medium
- Papaya—1 cup, cubed
- Peach—1 medium
- Pear—1 medium
- Plum—1 large
- Pomegranate seeds—½ cup
- Pumpkin—1 cup, cubed; ½ cup, mashed
- Raspberries—1 cup
- Strawberries—1 cup

HD-Friendly Fruits
Amount: After Start Strong, up to 1 serving per day as a *substitution* for 1 high-hydro fruit

HD-friendly fruits are higher in sugar than their high-hydro counterparts, and they don't have the same hydrophilic qualities. I like to get my clients used to eating the high-hydro fruits, which is why the 2-week Start Strong phase does not include HD-friendly ones. After Start Strong, you can have up to 1 serving of HD-friendly fruits per day in the serving size suggested.

- Banana—½ medium
- Cantaloupe—1 cup, cubed
- Cherries—1 cup (18)
- Grapes—1 cup (15)
- Honeydew melon—1 cup, cubed
- Pineapple—1 cup, cubed
- Watermelon—1 cup, cubed

Note: Please don't add these high-sugar fruits too soon! Whenever you can, make a high-hydro fruit choice.

Dried Fruits
Amount: Count toward HD-friendly fruit total

In dried fruits the water has been removed (no hydro!), which also means their sugars are concentrated. Since the following fruits are still high in HD fiber and nutrients, I consider them HD friendly. Sweet and portable, they make a great snack in the right portions.

- ○ Dried apricots—5 pieces
- ○ Dried mango—3 strips
- ○ Dried plums (prunes)—5 pieces
- ○ Dried figs—3 pieces

Hydro-Booster: Chia Seeds
Amount: 2 tablespoons of chia seeds or 6 tablespoons of Chia Gel per day

On the HD plan, chia seeds are strategically incorporated into your meals and snacks throughout the day. Using chia can be as simple as sprinkling the seeds on a salad or mixing Chia Gel (page 158) into a soup or smoothie. The hydro-boost from chia is especially helpful to stave off the hunger that makes you vulnerable to the Danishes brought in by a thoughtful coworker, the office vending machine, or the after-school cookie monster.

For example, my clients who are desperate to raid the cabinets at 3:00 p.m. help temper that impulse by having a hydro-booster at lunch. If by dinner you usually feel ravenous enough to eat the kitchen table, an afternoon snack with a hydro-booster makes good sense for you. Reviewing your food logs and hunger data can help you determine when you need that chia hydro-boost most.

I suggest you have a total of 2 tablespoons (6 teaspoons) of chia seeds or 6 tablespoons of the gel with at least one meal *and* one snack per day. Some clients love adding chia and regularly have 3 tablespoons a day, and that's fine.

For maximum satiety, break up the recommended daily amount over a total of at least one meal or snack per day. This means approximately 1 tablespoon of seeds or 3 tablespoons of gel each time. Remember—1 tablespoon of raw seeds equals 3 tablespoons of gel.

High-Hydro Proteins
Amount: Up to 4 servings of high-hydro proteins or HD-friendly proteins (see next section) per day

Beans, beans are good for your heart; the more you eat, the fuller you are! So that's a bit silly but true. Low in fat, high in HD fiber, and packed with protein, legumes are a great addition to your daily HD menu. The fiber in beans dissolves in water to trap bile acids in its gummy goo, which helps lower levels of LDL (bad) cholesterol. Not to mention that beans keep you satiated for hours.

The HD bean rule: Beans lead a triple life on the HD plan.

1. I love beans as a main source of protein! When you're not including an HD-friendly protein, such as chicken, as a main dish, beans (see full list below) count as a high-hydro protein. The serving is 1 cup whole or ½ cup mashed.
2. When you eat beans as a snack in between meals, they also count as a high-hydro protein. Here the serving size is ½ cup whole or ¼ cup mashed.
3. When you have beans in conjunction with an HD-friendly protein, they count as a high-hydro carb. The portion is decreased to ½ cup whole or ¼ cup mashed.

For example, if you're preparing 4 ounces of salmon with lentils and unlimited high-hydro vegetables for dinner, the lentils should be portioned to ½ cup and counted as a high-hydro carb. If lentils are your main source of protein (i.e., no salmon), then the portion would increase to 1 cup. If you prepared a salad filled with high-hydro vegetables and added 4 ounces of chicken breast, you could add ½ cup of beans and count them as a high-hydro carb.

However, if you are having unlimited high-hydro vegetables with hummus as a snack, the serving of hummus should be ¼ cup and you would count it as one of your high-hydro proteins.

I encourage my clients to enjoy their beans! If you like eating a bigger portion of beans as your main meal, just skip the HD-friendly protein.

- Adzuki beans
- Baby lima beans
- Bean spreads
- Black beans
- Black-eyed peas
- Cannellini beans
- Chickpeas
- Cowpeas
- Edamame
- Fava beans
- Great Northern beans

- Kidney beans (light or dark)
- Large lima beans (also called butter beans)
- Lentils
- Mung beans
- Peas
- Navy beans
- Pink beans
- Pinto beans
- Soybeans
- White beans

HD-Friendly Proteins
Amount: Up to 4 servings of HD-friendly proteins or high-hydro proteins (see previous section) per day

Unfortunately, many dieters overportion protein foods and eat them with absolutely no high-hydro foods on the side. This leads to a quick drop in your satisfaction levels on the Hunger Determination Scale. HD-friendly proteins should be consumed with hearty portions of high-hydro vegetables in order to get the most satisfaction and satiety. A serving of HD-friendly protein is 4 ounces for women and 6 ounces for men unless otherwise noted.

The menus in the next chapter will give you great-tasting protein and veggie recipes and combinations to try, like Chia-Crusted Salmon with Zucchini "Fettuccine" (pages 212 and 205, respectively). I included egg substitutes to have on hand for busy mornings.

- Chicken breast
- Clams
- Cod
- Crabmeat
- Eggs—5 egg whites or 1 egg and 2 egg whites
- Flounder
- Greek yogurt (6 ounces)
- Grouper
- Halibut
- Lobster
- Mahi mahi
- Mussels
- Ocean perch
- Orange roughy
- Rainbow trout
- Salmon, wild
- Sardines
- Scallops*
- Sea bass
- Shrimp*
- Squid
- Swordfish
- Tempeh
- Tofu
- Tuna
- Turkey breast

*How many? Buy a pound of shrimp or scallops and divide by four for 4 ounces. Usually this translates as 5 to 6 pieces, but it varies.

High-Hydro Carbohydrates
Amount: Up to 2 servings per day; 1 additional serving added in the Soaring in HD phase

Unlike some weight-loss programs, the HD plan does *not* eliminate carbohydrates because whole, unrefined grains are fiber rich and full of nutrients, and they help us feel satiated. They also provide energy and help prevent the binge episodes that are common when carbohydrates are eliminated from our diets completely.

The following is a list of high-fiber, highly satisfying carbs that have exceptional hydrophilic qualities. Eat at least 1 and up to 2 servings of high-hydro carbs per day; you can add another serving of carbs once you have reached the Soaring in HD phase. A serving is considered to be ½ cup cooked unless otherwise noted.

- Acorn squash—½ cup, cubed
- Amaranth
- Barley
- Beans from the high-hydro protein list (if eaten with an HD-friendly protein)
- Brown rice
- Buckwheat
- Butternut squash—½ cup, cubed
- Farro
- Oat bran
- Oatmeal—½ cup rolled (old fashioned); ¼ cup steel-cut
- Parsnips
- Quinoa
- Rye berries
- Sweet potato, with skin—½ cup cubed or ½ medium potato

HD-Friendly Carbohydrates
Amount: Up to 1 serving per day as a *substitution* for 1 high-hydro carb

Whole grain, high-fiber breads, cereals, crackers, and wraps can be a part of your HD plan, but they don't have the same hydrophilic qualities that the high-hydro carbs have. I encourage you to always have at least one high-hydro carbohydrate, like oats or a sweet potato.

But sometimes you just need a grab-and-go carb that you can put or spread something on, or crunch. I know this, which is why I have HD-friendly carb rules for you.

Combine these carbs with high-hydro veggies and fruits and your hydro-booster chia seeds to enhance satiety.

- Breads: 100 calories or less per serving; 3 grams of fiber or more*
- Cereals: 150 calories or less per serving; 5 grams of fiber or more, 6 grams or less of sugar
- Chips, snack foods: 100 calories or less per serving; 3 grams of fiber or more

- Crackers: 100 calories or less per serving; 3 grams of fiber or more
- Ezekiel 4:9 whole grain sesame (1 slice)
- Pepperidge Farm 7-Grain Deli Flat
- Popcorn (air popped): 3 cups
- Wraps: 100 calories or less per serving; 3 grams of fiber or more

*Sometimes it's not easy to find breads and wraps that fit the above criteria. My favorite wraps are La Tortilla Factory's low-carb wraps, Tumaro's Low in Carb Multi Grain Tortillas, and Food for Life 4:9 Ezekiel Bread.

Decision Nutrition Chia Bagels and Chia Chips fit the criteria, too. The kicker is that they have the hydro-boost of chia seeds built in so they keep you full for hours. My clients love them because—hey—who doesn't like to nosh on a bagel or some chips and still lose weight!?

HD-Friendly MUFA (Monounsaturated Fatty Acid) Amount: Once a day only as a snack or added to a meal

First, a primer on potentially helpful dietary fat. The two main types are:

Monounsaturated fat. This fat is found in a variety of foods and oils. Eating foods rich in monounsaturated fats (MUFAs) may decrease your risk of heart disease by improving your blood cholesterol levels. Studies demonstrate that MUFAs can lower total (serum) and LDL (bad) cholesterol levels while maintaining or increasing HDL (good) cholesterol. MUFAs may also help normalize blood clotting. In addition, MUFAs have been shown to help control insulin and blood sugar levels, which can be especially helpful if you have type 2 diabetes.

WHY GREEK YOGURT?

A large amount of the lactose-containing whey has been strained out, so Greek yogurt is thicker than regular yogurt. It's also higher in protein and lower in carbs. And since all of the carbohydrates naturally found in yogurt come from lactose, a lower-carb yogurt means a lower-lactose yogurt. Many lactose-intolerant people can tolerate Greek yogurt, which is why I allow it even in the Start Strong phase.

Polyunsaturated fat. This fat is found mostly in plant-based foods and oils. Evidence shows that eating foods rich in polyunsaturated fats improves blood cholesterol levels, potentially lowering your risk of heart disease. These fats may also help decrease the risk of type 2 diabetes. Omega-3 fatty acids, one type of polyunsaturated fat, may benefit your heart and arteries especially. These omega-3s, which are found in some types of fatty fish, may also protect against irregular heartbeats and help lower blood pressure.

Key to remember: Unlike butter or lard, monounsaturated and polyunsaturated fats are liquid at room temperature. Think olive oil, safflower oil, peanut oil, and corn oil.

I love the MUFA foods on the following list because they are satisfying and healthy. The problem is that many people overindulge in these foods, and they contain a lot of calories and fat. My male clients will sometimes eat an entire 12-ounce bag of almonds because they are watching their weight. That bag tallies in at around 1,968 calories and 172 grams of healthy fat! That is too much, no matter how healthy. The same goes for avocados, which weigh in at 322 calories and 30 grams of fat for a medium-size one. Remember, you can gain weight on healthy foods, too. If you have one-quarter of an avocado in your salad, don't add nuts!

While comparatively high in calories and fat per serving, nuts, nut butters, and seeds pack a nutritional punch and are also very satisfying, making them a great snack when eaten in moderation. Chia Gel (page 158) can help hydro-stretch the amount of nut butter being used, so you get a larger portion (see note on page 225).

You can pick from this list once a day as a snack or meal addition. Look at snack examples in Chapter 11 to see how to couple these HD-friendly fats with high-hydro foods.

- ○ Almond butter (1 tablespoon) or chia almond butter (2 tablespoons)
- ○ Almonds (15 or 100-calorie snack pack)
- ○ Avocado (¼ of a whole)
- ○ Olives (15)
- ○ Peanut butter, natural (1 tablespoon) or chia peanut butter (see note on page 225) (2 tablespoons)
- ○ Pistachios (24 or 100-calorie snack pack)
- ○ Pumpkin seeds (¼ cup)
- ○ Sesame seeds (¼ cup)
- ○ Sunflower seeds (¼ cup)
- ○ Walnuts (6 halves)

ADDITIONAL HD FOODS

Seaweeds

Amount: Unlimited

Seaweeds *love* water, so it's only natural that a hydrophilic diet would consider seaweed a top choice on its list of recommended foods! Seaweeds are not technically vegetables but are often called sea vegetables. They are mostly composed of hydrophilic fiber (think about the viscous texture of the seaweed you've seen in the ocean). And they also contain calcium, iron, vitamin A, niacin, and significant amounts of iodine.

If you have never considered eating seaweed, or the thought grosses you out, know that they have great flavor, too, and many cultures recognize them for the nutritious, delicious food they are. In fact, seaweeds are integral to Japanese cuisine; if you've ever eaten a California roll or had miso soup, I can pretty much guarantee you've eaten seaweed. Another popular seaweed product is roasted seaweed, and these "chips" are unlimited on the HD plan.

Here is a list of high-hydrophilic seaweeds and descriptions.

- Arame comes in thin black threads and is mild in flavor.
- Dulse can add a baconlike saltiness and crunch without the fat and cholesterol!
- Kelp noodles are made from kelp, seaweed salt, and water. They can be eaten raw or cooked and have a neutral taste that suits a variety of purposes, including salads, stir-fries, soups, and casseroles. They are fat free, gluten free, low in carbs and calories, and provide a rich source of trace minerals, including iodine.
- Kombu is used in traditional Japanese broths, like dashi. It is a hydrophilic wonder and even makes your bean dishes more digestible.
- Agar (also called agar-agar) is, at 80 percent soluble fiber, the most hydrophilic of the seaweeds. Dissolved in hot water and cooled, it becomes gelatinous, so vegans often use agar instead of animal protein–based gelatin.
- Nori comes in a flat sheet and is used in sushi. I encourage my clients to use nori as a sandwich wrap, just as you would a tortilla.
- Wakame expands and softens when cooked, so it's often used in soups (like miso soup).

I urge you to experiment with different types of seaweed. You can add wakame to soup and bean dishes, make arame salad, or use nori to roll up turkey or bean fillings. You can even make "chocolate mousse" with agar.

Shirataki Noodles
Amount: Unlimited

You may have heard of—or already be using—shirataki noodles. In the past few years, they've become well known as a dieter's friend, and you can have unlimited quantities of them on the HD plan. Shirataki noodles are made from the root of the konnyaku potato, a plant grown throughout Asia. This plant is rich in glucomannan, which is a very water-absorbent fiber. The noodles don't contain any other nutrients, but they "phill up" dishes, like soups and stir-fries, to help keep you satisfied.

Shirataki noodles are sometimes fortified with tofu (tofu shirataki noodles), which gives them a slightly heftier texture as well as adding a bit of protein and carbs. With or without tofu, shirataki noodles are both unlimited on the HD plan and generally available in supermarkets. You can usually find them in the refrigerated section under the names Konjac, Skinny Shirataki Noodles, Tofu Shirataki, etc. Follow the package instructions on rinsing and parboiling them.

Herbs, Spices, Condiments, and Other Flavorings
Amount: Unlimited

Alliums and Herbs

While some of these are available dried, I recommend buying them fresh for the best flavor. Alliums—basically the onion and garlic family—come in many different flavors. For a healthy variety, experiment with leeks, scallions, or any kind you're not used to eating regularly.

- ○ Basil
- ○ Capers
- ○ Chervil
- ○ Chives
- ○ Cilantro
- ○ Dill
- ○ Garlic
- ○ Leeks
- ○ Lemongrass
- ○ Marjoram
- ○ Mint
- ○ Oregano
- ○ Parsley
- ○ Rosemary
- ○ Sage
- ○ Scallions
- ○ Shallots
- ○ Tarragon
- ○ Thyme

Spices

On top of adding flavor to your meals, spices also add a wealth of micronutrients. Remember, though, that spices left in your cabinet for more than a year are best chucked, honestly.

- ○ Allspice
- ○ Anise
- ○ Bay leaf
- ○ Black pepper
- ○ Caraway
- ○ Cardamom
- ○ Celery seed
- ○ Chicory
- ○ Chili powder
- ○ Cinnamon
- ○ Cloves
- ○ Coriander
- ○ Crab-boil seasoning
- ○ Cumin
- ○ Garlic powder
- ○ Ground ginger
- ○ Ground red pepper
- ○ Mustard seed
- ○ Nutmeg
- ○ Onion powder
- ○ Paprika
- ○ Pumpkin pie spice
- ○ Red-pepper flakes
- ○ Salt substitutes
- ○ Seasoning blends (no added sugar or salt)
- ○ Turmeric

Condiments and Flavorings

The following condiments and flavorings are unlimited daily unless otherwise noted.

- ○ Extracts (like vanilla, peppermint, almond)
- ○ Horseradish
- ○ Hot-pepper sauce
- ○ Lemon and lime wedges or juice
- ○ Mustard (choose varieties with no sweeteners added)
- ○ Salsa
- ○ Stevia—One quick note here: On the HD plan, cravings for sweets are satisfied with fruits and natural sweeteners, like stevia. Some brands of stevia are: Truvia, Nu Stevia, and Sweet Leaf. If you're addicted to the kick of artificial sugar alternatives, like saccharin or aspartame, believe me when I tell you that my clients have much more success when they eliminate these products from their diets. I go into this topic in more detail in Chapter 7.
- ○ Vinegars
- ○ Wasabi

WHAT ABOUT COOKING SPRAYS?

I keep them in my pantry for cooking egg whites or giving my high-hydro veggies a spritz when I want them roasted. But, just so you know, there is a misconception around these sprays.

If they are oil, how are they calorie and fat free? Tricky advertising is the answer. If a product contains fewer than 5 calories or 0.5 gram of fat in a single serving, the company is legally allowed to claim the product has zero calories and is fat free.

One serving of cooking spray equals a ⅓-second spray (which wouldn't coat much of anything).

A 1-second squirt is usually 7 to 10 calories and 1 gram of fat.

So don't get spray-happy. Spray for 4 seconds maximum and you're done. That's your time limit. If you use an olive oil sprayer or mister, it's around 10 seconds.

While the following flavorings are delicious and healthful, they should be used sparingly as they generally contain sugar, fat, or added salt. The following are the amounts alloted per day.

Bragg Liquid Aminos—1 tablespoon

Miso paste—1 teaspoon

Reduced-sodium soy sauce—1 tablespoon

Reduced-sodium tamari—1 tablespoon

Sauerkraut, reduced sodium—½ cup

Tomato paste—1 tablespoon

Tomato sauce—½ cup; 5 grams of sugar or less

Unsweetened cocoa powder— 2 teaspoons (Believe it or not, it has fiber!)

HD-Friendly Liquids

Water—There's nothing like a tall glass of water to flush out your system, help digestion, moisturize your skin, and keep you energized! Drink at least six to eight glasses per day. (You can include lemon water and herbal teas in this tally.)

Unsweetened almond milk (original or vanilla), 1¼ cups—I prefer almond milk, but other milk substitutes are unsweetened coconut milk (1¼ cups), unsweetened rice milk (1 cup), or unsweetened soy milk (1 cup).

Coffee (with almond milk; no sugar, half-and-half, artificial sweeteners, or creamers added)—No more than 2 cups and not as a substitute for food!

Reduced-sodium broth (chicken, beef, vegetable, fish)

Sparkling water (add flavor with lemon or lime)

Teas—All types of teas are allowed on the HD plan, although because of the caffeine it's better to drink herbal tea. Nettle and dandelion teas are my top picks. They have detoxifying properties and are natural diuretics, so these teas help keep the hydro-flow going and diminish bloat. Of course, there's no such thing as a tea that will make you lose weight. But I do believe that tea breaks are relaxing, and while you drink yours, you can refresh yourself and remember why you are on this HD journey.

THE IF LIST

As mentioned earlier, *IF* is an acronym for *infrequent foods*. Desserts, fried foods, alcohol, refined carbs, cheeses, chips-and-dips—these are all foods that, quite frankly, aren't very good for you. All people have their weaknesses. I personally have a wicked sweet tooth, and my downfalls happen to be black-and-white cookies, Duncan Hines frosting, and Twizzlers. Yours might be red wine or a hunk of cheese or french fries or your mother's homemade pasta with Bolognese sauce. So I know I can't tell you to cut these foods out forever or you might close the book on me!

What I *will* say is that in order to live in HD, you'll have to decide what *place* these foods will have in your life. If you want to lose weight and maintain your weight loss, that place cannot be "all you want, whenever you want." If that blissful fairytale land existed, you wouldn't be reading this book. Living in HD means making the decision to eat or drink your IFs *occasionally*, and only IF you will truly savor them.

I highly recommend that you go without your IFs for as long as possible; at the very least, skip all IFs during the Start Strong phase. The longer you go without your IFs, the more quickly you'll see weight loss results, and the more psychologically prepared you will be to make the critical changes in your thinking around IFs.

It's up to you to decide how long you can last without your IFs. Some of my clients stick to the HD food lists in this chapter for the entire 12-week program or longer. Others crave that glass of wine or piece of cheese from the very beginning and can't wait to have it back. In Chapter 7 you'll get to explore your own IFs. You'll learn *why* they are IFs and HD tips and tricks on how to keep them "in their place."

Remember, it's all about decisions.

For now, as you start learning to live in HD, know that the following IF categories are not included in the first phase, Start Strong.

Alcohol

Artificial sweeteners

Butter and margarine

Canned foods with added sugar or salt

Cheese

Cow's milk, cream, and ice cream

Fried foods

Processed foods with added sugar or salt (if it can spend months or even years in the cabinet and still be edible, avoid it)

Pizza

Red meat or processed meat (like bacon, ham, sausage)

Refined sweets (like cakes, candy, cookies, pastries, pies)

Salt (the free-handed shake)

Snack foods (chips, pretzels, basically anything in a bag)

White pasta and white bread

DIANE, 44, *Lost 20 Pounds*

Before HD: Over the last few years, my weight had been slowly increasing by a few pounds a year. Before I met Keren, I was certain that if I went on a plan to lose weight, I'd inevitably feel hungry and deprived. How wrong I was! Keren gave me food options and ideas that may seem obvious but had never occurred to me before.

Starting strong: I consistently food-logged every day for the first 12 weeks so I could honestly see what I was eating and how this worked with my lifestyle.

New foods: Pomegranate seeds. Grilled rosemary salmon and green beans. Crudités. Bean dips. I don't ever feel the need to eat something that may give me a moment of pleasure but won't satisfy me for very long.

Unexpected bonus: I only drink water or seltzer now, which I love!

Lesson learned: When I go on vacation, I bring some of my favorite foods with me if they are easy to transport.

New mantra: Feeling in control of your decisions is key. You should eat food because it is healthy and satisfying not because it is sitting in front of you. You need to be thoughtful about it.

Sustaining in HD: I am more careful about choosing which foods I really want to eat as opposed to simply indulging in foods that just look tempting. Also, with desserts, I've learned that eating a couple of bites has the same benefit as eating an entire piece.

What's next: Food is a big part of my Jewish culture, and I am now able to embrace big, festive, holiday meals because I understand better about portions and what foods are more filling. I feel much happier that I can continue my busy social calendar—going to parties and hosting holiday and Sabbath meals at my house—without worrying anymore about the effect it will have on my weight.

Inspiring words: The HD plan is designed to help you make good decisions—no matter what time of day it is or where you are. It teaches you what foods work for you and make you happy, satisfied, and full for longer.

WHAT? NO OLIVE OIL?

Olive oil is famous for its heart-healthy benefits. It's a culinary star; its name practically appears in lights in so many recipes and diet plans. But like nuts and avocado, olive oil has got to be called out for its fat and calories. It may be heart healthy, but that doesn't mean it's "free"!

At 120 calories and 14 grams of fat per tablespoon, olive oil can easily be one of the reasons why your pants fit tight. I love the example of typical sautéed garlic-and-oil spinach ordered at a restaurant. You heap it on your plate because, well, you're watching your weight and trying to be healthy! However, I can almost guarantee that in that beautiful green mound there's a lot more than a single tablespoon of olive oil. Try three or four! That adds up to almost 500 calories.

Please—I beg you—don't do it! If you're going to pack on the pounds, at least enjoy yourself and have a dessert like tiramisu. I just don't want you eating 500-calorie spinach! It really upsets me. Please, please watch the heart-healthy olive oil (or any other oil, for that matter).

Order it steamed. A cup of steamed spinach has 40 calories and none of the fat.

6

START STRONG IN HD— DAILY CHECKLISTS AND MENUS

"Before you can think out of the box, you have to start with a box."

—TWYLA THARP

Decisions, decisions, decisions. So far I've talked a lot about decisions, so you'll be happy to know that in this chapter I'm going to make it easy for you. In the following pages, you will find:

- The HD "Cheat Sheet" plate
- A 14-day HD Start Strong menu plan
- The top five HD-friendly kitchen tools
- Keren's reminders
- 12 weeks of decisions for Maya the Busy Mama
- HD freebies

Why do you need a "cheat sheet"? When I have a new client, I arrange fake plastic foods on a plate to illustrate correct portion sizes. Many times this demonstration gets a laugh (or grunt) from whoever is sitting across from me because, well, it seems so elementary.

But truth be told, all of my clients have said that the plastic foods presentation delivered a valuable lesson. So I've tried to re-create this experience here for you. The HD Cheat Sheet plate (below) is designed to make all the portion rules easier to follow.

In fact, these guidelines are *especially* valuable when dining out. It is difficult to come across a restaurant these days that doesn't serve oversize portions, so you have to be vigilant. If handed a chicken breast the size of your forearm, remember the plate guidelines and take half of it home. See page 158 for high-hydro carb serving sizes.

Cheat Sheet Plate

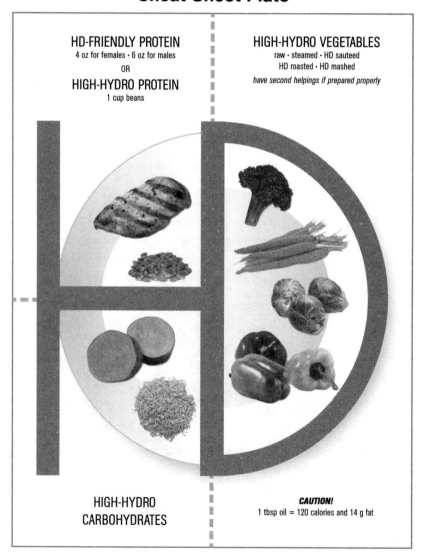

EASING INTO START STRONG

As your nutrition coach throughout this process, it's very important to me that you *actually follow the HD plan guidelines every day.* After a week or so on the plan, most of my clients settle into a pattern. They find their favorite breakfasts, lunches, and dinners, which makes planning meals for the week much easier.

Research shows that people who successfully slim down and stay at their new weights tend to eat comparable things each day.[1] I find that clients who really want to change it up every day get discouraged quickly because being exciting requires a lot of thought and prep! But it's fine to be boring and eat oatmeal nearly every day. *I believe living in HD is frustration free.* The key is to have your favorite go-to meals and introduce one or two new dishes weekly. And the easier it is to whip up your meals, the more likely it is you will stick to the plan. If you enjoy a new dish, just incorporate it into your rotation.

At first it may feel unnatural for some of you to be so proactive about food shopping, preparing, and logging. However, once you get into a groove, like all my successful clients, you'll soon find your favorites.

Many of my clients express concerns about getting all the nutrients they need on the HD plan. If you're incorporating your high-hydro vegetables and fruits throughout the day and you remember your daily chia seeds, you will hit your Recommended Dietary Allowances for sure!

14-DAY HD START STRONG MENU PLAN

Here's a 14-day suggested menu—just as a guide. It is composed of many of my favorite HD meals, and you can find the recipes for them in Chapter 11. You can change the order of the days, repeat a meal or snack you like, and use the core foods lists to change a suggestion. (For example, if 1 cup of raspberries—a high-hydro fruit—is listed and you'd rather have 1 cup of strawberries, go for it!)

You basically want to get into the mind-set of loosely devising menus before the start of each new week so grocery shopping and meal prep are easy.

I have definitely come to realize that complicated Julia Childesque meals equate to HD noncompliance. And this wisdom is reflected in the following plan because you actually have to *do* the plan in order to live in HD. Meal assembly using the Ultimate HD Salad (page 161) and the HD "Cheat Sheet" (page 90) are meant to help you keep it simple. They give you the power to decide, plus they are quick!

I listed the category each meal falls under to make it easier for you to use the food lists in Chapter 5. Remember: As long as you follow the principles, you are starting strong.

DAY 1

**The guidelines for building the Ultimate HD Salad start on page 161. The way I laid it out, you get to choose the high-hydro vegetables you like. Check it out!*

***This is a meal you would build using the HD "Cheat Sheet" plate on page 90: 1/2 plate of high-hydro vegetables, 1/4 plate of protein, and 1/4 plate of a high-hydro carb. It's a great way not to stress the "What's for dinner?" dilemma. In Chapter 10, I give simple guidelines on how to cook the high-hydro grains and beans and how to prepare high-hydro vegetables the HD way.*

BREAKFAST	LUNCH	DINNER
Quick Chia Oatmeal (page 173) *high-hydro carb, hydro-booster* **1 cup raspberries** *high-hydro fruit*	**Ultimate HD Salad (page 161)** *high-hydro vegetable** **1 tablespoon chia seeds** *hydro-booster* **Choice of any Good Decisions Dressing (pages 189–192) or free condiment (page 82)** **Lemon Grilled Chicken (page 209)** *HD-friendly protein*	**Good Decisions Soup (page 195)** *high-hydro vegetable* **HD "Cheat Sheet"** *high-hydro vegetable, high-hydro/HD-friendly protein, high-hydro carb***
A.M. SNACK	**P.M. SNACK**	**NIGHTTIME SNACK**
1 apple *high-hydro fruit* **15 almonds** *HD-friendly MUFA*	**HD Crudité (page 165)** *high-hydro vegetable* **1/4 cup Chickpea Spread (page 183) or store-bought hummus (I love the hummus brand by Good Neighbors Simply Zero.)** *high-hydro protein*	**Free Frozen Fruit Skewer (page 222)**

DAY 2

BREAKFAST	LUNCH	DINNER
Eggsellent Omelet (page 178) *HD-friendly protein, high-hydro vegetable, hydro-booster*	**HD "Cheat Sheet"** *high-hydro carb, high-hydro/HD-friendly protein, high-hydro vegetable**	**Asparagus and Artichoke Salad (page 187)** *high-hydro vegetable* **Lemon Grilled Chicken (page 209)** *HD-friendly protein*
A.M. SNACK	**P.M. SNACK**	**NIGHTTIME SNACK**
1 pear *high-hydro fruit* **1 tablespoon almond butter** *HD-friendly MUFA*	**Berry Parfait (page 219)** *HD-friendly protein, high-hydro fruit, hydro-booster*	**HD Popcorn (page 229)** *HD-friendly carb*

**This is the same concept as the plate, but you use a big bowl to build your meal. Picture three layers: a high-hydro carbohydrate on the bottom, a high-hydro/HD-friendly protein in the middle, and a lot of high-hydro vegetables on top.*

I keep the layers plain and simple, and then add some Miso Dressing (page 191) or a tablespoon of Bragg Liquid Aminos or reduced-sodium tamari. One-quarter cup of reduced-sugar tomato sauce works, too!

CARB FAKE-OUTS!

On the HD plan, you can have two carbohydrates a day from the approved lists. However, there will be times when you feel like you want more or you just don't want to use up a carb yet.

Good news: You can fake a carb with these carblike tastes and textures:

- Spaghetti squash
- Cabbage spaghetti
- Shirataki noodles
- Mashed Turnips (page 201)
- Zucchini "Fettuccine" (page 205)
- Nori used as a wrap
- Collard green used as a wrap
- Kelp noodles

DAY 3

BREAKFAST	LUNCH	DINNER
While-You-Sleep Chia Oatmeal (page 174) *high-hydro carb, hydro-booster* **1 cup strawberries** *high-hydro fruit*	**Build a Wrap (page 164); with a collard green leaf and 4 ounces fresh turkey or chicken from the deli counter (house)** *high-hydro vegetable, HD-friendly protein**	**Chia-Crusted Salmon (page 212)** *HD-friendly protein, hydro-booster* **HD roasted vegetables (see page 167 for cooking tips)** *high-hydro vegetable* **Sweet Potato Roast (page 204)** *high-hydro carb*
A.M. SNACK	**P.M. SNACK**	**NIGHTTIME SNACK**
Jicama-Nut Sandwich (page 225) *high-hydro vegetable, HD-friendly MUFA, hydro-booster*	**Yogurt Dip (page 182)** *HD-friendly protein* **HD Crudité (page 165)** *high-hydro vegetable*	**Vanilla Agar Pudding (page 220)** **1 cup raspberries** *high-hydro fruit*

**This is a meal that also enables you to make your own decisions. You can use an HD-friendly wrap, like La Tortilla Factory's low-carb ones, and fill it with your choice of HD-friendly protein or high-hydro protein, like a bean spread. The key is to load up the wrap with high-hydro sandwich fillers. See page 164 for wrap guidelines and suggestions. On this day, a carb fake-out is used so you can have a high-hydro carb at dinner.*

DAY 4

BREAKFAST	LUNCH	DINNER
Microwave Chia Egg Soufflé (page 179) *HD-friendly protein, high-hydro vegetable, hydro-booster* **1 Decision Nutrition Chia Bagel** *HD-friendly carb, hydro-booster*	**Vegetable-Chia Miso Soup (page 198)** *high-hydro vegetable, hydro-booster* **Salmon Salad Nori Wrap (page 214)** *HD-friendly protein, high-hydro vegetable, hydro-booster*	**Broccoli Soup (page 193)** *high-hydro vegetable* **Balsamic Chicken (page 208)** *HD-friendly protein, high-hydro vegetable, hydro-booster* **½ cup cooked brown rice** *high-hydro carb*
A.M. SNACK	**P.M. SNACK**	**NIGHTTIME SNACK**
1 orange *high-hydro fruit* **24 pistachios** *HD-friendly MUFA*	**Chia Smoothie (page 225)** *high-hydro fruit, hydro-booster*	**Lemon Custard Agar Pudding (page 220)**

DAY 5

BREAKFAST	LUNCH	DINNER
Barley Breakfast (page 175) with 1 tablespoon chia seeds *high-hydro carb, hydro-booster* **1 cup blackberries** *high-hydro fruit*	**Ultimate HD Salad with Greek Flair (page 163)** *high-hydro vegetable* **1 cup chickpeas** *high-hydro protein* **8 Decision Nutrition Chia Chips** *HD-friendly carb, hydro-booster*	**Lemon Grilled Chicken (page 209)** *HD-friendly protein* **HD sautéed vegetables (see page 166 for cooking tips)** *high-hydro vegetable* **Mashed Turnips (page 201)** *high-hydro vegetable*
A.M. SNACK	**P.M. SNACK**	**NIGHTTIME SNACK**
Avocado Eggs (page 230) *HD-friendly protein, HD-friendly MUFA*	**Nori Vegetable Wrap (page 227)** *high-hydro vegetable*	**Raspberry-Cacao Sorbet (page 233)** *high-hydro fruit, hydro-booster*

DAY 6

BREAKFAST	LUNCH	DINNER
Brussels Egg Scramble (page 176) *HD-friendly protein, high-hydro vegetable* **½ grapefruit** *high-hydro fruit*	**Ultimate HD Salad with Asian Flair (page 164)** *high-hydro vegetable* **6 large steamed shrimp** *HD-friendly protein* **1 orange** *high-hydro fruit*	**Turkey Chili (page 199)** *HD-friendly protein, high-hydro carb*
A.M. SNACK	**P.M. SNACK**	**NIGHTTIME SNACK**
1 Decision Nutrition Chia Bagel with Chia-Raspberry Smash (page 185) and 1 tablespoon almond butter *HD-friendly carb, HD-friendly MUFA, hydro-booster*	**Dill Yogurt Dip with Chia Gel (page 182)** *HD-friendly protein, hydro-booster* **Kale Chips (page 226)** *high-hydro vegetable*	**Good Decisions Vanilla Chia Pudding (page 222)** *hydro-booster* **1 cup blueberries** *high-hydro fruit*

Don't forget: If you have an HD-friendly protein and a high-hydro protein together, the high-hydro one counts as a carbohydrate. This is to keep portions in check for the day. If you want to save a carbohydrate, prepare the Turkey Chili without turkey and it will count as a protein.

DAY 7

BREAKFAST	LUNCH	DINNER
Quick Cacao Chia Oatmeal (page 173) *high-hydro carb, hydro-booster* **1 cup strawberries** *high-hydro fruit*	**HD Black Bean Burrito (To make, combine the Black Bean Dip on page 184 with the Build a Wrap on page 164)** *HD-friendly carb, high-hydro protein*	**Ultimate HD Salad (page 161)** *high-hydro vegetable* **Scallop Stir-Fry Shirataki (page 217)** *HD-friendly protein, high-hydro vegetable*
A.M. SNACK	**P.M. SNACK**	**NIGHTTIME SNACK**
HD Crudité (page 165) *high-hydro vegetable* **Edamame Dip (page 185)** *high-hydro protein, hydro-booster*	**1 peach** *high-hydro fruit* **15 almonds** *HD-friendly MUFA*	**Free Frozen Fruit Skewer (page 222)** **0% plain Greek yogurt for dipping (6 ounces)** *HD-friendly protein*

DAY 8

BREAKFAST	LUNCH	DINNER
Swiss Chard Mini Frittata (page 180) *HD-friendly protein, high-hydro vegetable* **1 apple** *high-hydro fruit*	**Good Decisions Soup (page 195)** *high-hydro vegetable* **Build a Wrap (page 164)** *HD-friendly carb, high-hydro/HD-friendly protein, high-hydro vegetable*	**Cinnamon Chicken (page 208)** *HD-friendly protein, hydro-booster* **½ cup cooked amaranth** *high-hydro carb* **High-hydro veggies of your choice (choose prep style from Chapter 10)** *high-hydro vegetable*
A.M. SNACK	**P.M. SNACK**	**NIGHTTIME SNACK**
Nutmeg Pumpkin Mash with Walnuts (page 223) *high-hydro fruit, HD-friendly MUFA, hydro-booster*	**Nori Vegetable Hummus Wrap (page 227)** *high-hydro protein, high-hydro vegetable*	**Lemon Custard Agar Pudding (page 220)**

DAY 9

BREAKFAST	LUNCH	DINNER
Quick Chia Oatmeal (page 173) with Chia-Raspberry Smash (page 185) *high-hydro carb, hydro-booster* **Topped with almonds** *HD-friendly MUFA*	**Ultimate HD Salad with Italian Flair (page 163)** *high-hydro vegetable* **HD Tuna Salad (page 215)** *HD-friendly protein, high-hydro vegetable*	**Lima Bean–Okra Soup (page 197)** *high-hydro protein, high-hydro vegetable* **½ cup barley** *high-hydro carb*
A.M. SNACK	**P.M. SNACK**	**NIGHTTIME SNACK**
Berry Parfait (page 219) *HD-friendly protein, high-hydro fruit, hydro-booster*	**Chia Smoothie made with peaches (page 224)** *high-hydro fruit, hydro-booster*	**Roasted Chia Nori Strips (page 229)** *hydro-booster*

DAY 10

BREAKFAST	LUNCH	DINNER
Tofu Scrambler (page 181) *HD-friendly protein, high-hydro vegetable* **1 piece of rye bread** *HD-friendly carb*	**Ultimate HD Salad (page 161)** *high-hydro vegetable* **Lentil Soup (page 196)** *high-hydro protein, high hydro vegetable*	**Broccoli–Red Cabbage Slaw (page 188)** *high-hydro vegetable hydrobooster* **Spinach Turkey Burger (page 218)** *HD-friendly protein, high-hydro vegetable* **Parsnip Fries (page 202)** *high-hydro carb*
A.M. SNACK	**P.M. SNACK**	**NIGHTTIME SNACK**
1 orange *high-hydro fruit* **15 almonds** *HD-friendly MUFA*	**Berry Parfait (page 219)** *HD-friendly protein, high-hydro fruit, hydro-booster*	**Berry Mousse Agar Pudding (page 220)** *high-hydro fruit*

DAY 11

BREAKFAST	LUNCH	DINNER
While-You-Sleep Chia Oatmeal (page 174) *high-hydro carb, hydro-booster* **1 cup blueberries** *high-hydro fruit*	**HD "Cheat Sheet" (page 90)** *high-hydro/HD-friendly protein, high-hydro carb, high-hydro vegetable*	**Cabbage Spaghetti with Ground Chicken (page 210)** *HD-friendly protein, high-hydro vegetable*
A.M. SNACK	**P.M. SNACK**	**NIGHTTIME SNACK**
HD Crudité (page 165) *high-hydro vegetable* **½ cup White Bean Dip (page 184)** *high-hydro protein, hydro-booster*	**Good Decisions Soup (page 195)** *high-hydro vegetable*	**Good Decisions Cacao Chia Pudding (page 222)** *hydro-booster*

DAY 12

BREAKFAST	LUNCH	DINNER
Eggsellent Omelet (page 178) *HD-friendly protein, high-hydro vegetable, hydro-booster*	**Gazpacho Soup (page 194)** *high-hydro vegetable* **Crabmeat** *HD-friendly protein (4 ounces)*	**Balsamic Chicken (page 207)** *HD-friendly protein, high-hydro vegetable, hydro-booster* **HD Ratatouille (page 200)** *high-hydro vegetable* **Brown rice** *high-hydro carb (½ cup)*
A.M. SNACK	**P.M. SNACK**	**NIGHTTIME SNACK**
3 medium figs *high-hydro fruit* **2 tablespoons chia nut butter (page 183)** *HD-friendly MUFA, hydro-booster*	**HD Crudité (page 166)** *high-hydro vegetable* **Chickpea Spread (page 183)** *high-hydro protein, hydro-booster*	**HD Popcorn (page 229)** *HD-friendly carb*

DAY 13

BREAKFAST	LUNCH	DINNER
HD-friendly cereal (I love Barbara's Original Puffins) with almond milk *HD-friendly carb* **1 cup berries** *high-hydro fruit* **1 tablespoon chia seeds** *hydro-booster*	**Bean-Stuffed Acorn Squash (page 206)** *high-hydro protein, high-hydro vegetable, high-hydro carb, hydro-booster*	**Easy Fish (page 211)** *HD-friendly protein, high-hydro vegetable* **Zucchini "Fettuccine" (page 205)** *high-hydro vegetable*
A.M. SNACK	**P.M. SNACK**	**NIGHTTIME SNACK**
HD Crudité (page 165) *high-hydro vegetable* **Horseradish Yogurt Dip (page 182)** *HD-friendly protein*	**Poached Cinnamon Pear (page 232) topped with walnuts** *high-hydro fruit, HD-friendly MUFA*	**Berry Parfait (page 219)** *HD-friendly protein, high-hydro fruit, hydro-booster*

DAY 14

BREAKFAST	LUNCH	DINNER
Apple Cinnamon Oatmeal (page 172) with 1 tablespoon Chia seeds added in *high-hydro carb, high-hydro fruit, hydro-booster*	**Ultimate HD Salad with Latin Flair (page 164)** *high-hydro vegetable* **1 cup black beans** *high-hydro protein*	**Rosemary-Lemon Salmon (page 213)** *HD-friendly protein* **Sweet Potato Fries (page 204)** *high-hydro carb* **HD roasted vegetables (see page 167 for cooking tips)** *high-hydro vegetable*
A.M. SNACK	**P.M. SNACK**	**NIGHTTIME SNACK**
Nori Vegetable Wrap (page 227) *high-hydro vegetable*	**Peanut Butter Cup Agar Pudding (page 220)** *HD-friendly MUFA* **1 cup strawberries** *high-hydro fruit*	**Free Frozen Fruit Skewer (page 222)**

TOP FIVE HD-FRIENDLY KITCHEN TOOLS

All of these tools are used in the HD plan recipes and are great to have in your repertoire.

Hand blender. This is so much easier than using a regular blender for a lot of recipes! I use hand blenders for making soups (like the Broccoli Soup on page 193), for making Good Decisions Dressings (page 189), or for mashing beans or vegetables—anything you want to whip up. Just stick the ingredients in a bowl and turn it on. It's that simple.

Julienne cutter. This wonderful kitchen tool transforms high-hydro veggies into nice skinny strips, which are amazing in salads, as side dishes, or as sandwich fillers. Zucchini, carrots, jicama, and yellow squash all work, and you can use julienned zucchini and yellow squash as fake-out carbs. Check out the Zucchini "Fettuccine" recipe on page 205.

Mason jars. I always like to have mason jars on hand. They are perfect for storing your Chia Gel (page 158) or Chia-Raspberry Smash (page 185). These concoctions stay fresh for 2 weeks in the jars!

Ramekins. I love my ramekins! They come in different sizes: The 6-ouncers are great for any of the agar puddings (page 220), the Nutmeg Pumpkin Mash with Walnuts (page 223), or the chia puddings (page 222); and you can stock up on the 8-ouncers for cooking your Microwave Chia Egg Soufflé (page 179). Ramekins are just good to have on hand.

Steamer basket. If you don't own a steamer basket, you *must* get one immediately. Steaming high-hydro veggies is an HD must. I steam everything—even fish, chicken, and tofu. You name it, it's been in my basket. But steaming is truly great for high-hydro veggies; just throw them in and you will be HD satiated for hours. Check out the unlimited condiment list on page 82 for ways to add flavor, or top veggies with your choice of Good Decisions Dressings (page 189).

KEREN'S REMINDERS

The following weekly and daily to-do lists will help keep you organized. They are intended to serve as a quick reference of the important tasks that will help you achieve HD success.

Weekly

- ○ Stick to the weekly weigh-in day and time you have chosen, and always use the same scale (the one at the gym may say something different than your bathroom scale).
- ○ Record your weight on your weekly weight-tracking report provided at decisionnutrition.com.
- ○ Fill out a weekly goals sheet to remind yourself what you will focus on for the week. (See page 242 or decisionnutrition.com)
- ○ Wash, cut, and prep the fruits and vegetables you plan to use for the week. Check out Chapter 10 for high-hydro veggie prep options and inspiration. Store what you decide on in clear glass or plastic containers for easy access. If you can see it, you will eat it. (Warning! This is true for kids as well. If you have bright high-hydro vegetables or fruits displayed in the fridge, they may be gone before you get to them. Kids will eat what they see, too, so this can be a family-wide life-changer.)
- ○ Read over the dressing recipes on pages 189 to 192 and pick one to keep on hand for the week. (Store the dressing in a glass mason jar.)
- ○ Make a list of HD foods to get at the market.
- ○ If you've added IFs (infrequent foods) to your diet, note how they have affected your weight progress.
- ○ Make a soup for the week and keep it in the fridge. My favorite is the Good Decisions Soup on page 195!
- ○ Make your Chia Gel (page 158) and put it in a glass mason jar in the fridge (lasts up to 2 weeks).
- ○ Try a recipe out of your comfort zone once during the week. It may even get added to your daily go-to meal or snack options.
- ○ Remember, every week is a new beginning. Evaluate your progress; note the good decisions you made the week before. Reward yourself with a noncaloric treat—a bath, a massage, or some mindless reality TV.

- Address the bad decisions of the week before in your weekly goals sheet. Remember, a week is just a step in a long journey. The results are worth the climb.
- Eat mindfully and live decisively.

Daily

- Drink warm lemon water upon rising. It is good for digestion and reminds you that this is a fresh new day.
- Use the Hunger Determination Scale. Every day you should be more aware of what your body is telling you. Are you hungry? Stressed? Bored? Lonely? Become aware.
- Fill out your food logs.
- Look over the list of free snacks (page 106). These are limitless healthy snacks to diminish hunger pangs throughout the day.
- Eat breakfast!
- Use your hydro-boosting chia seeds!
- Refer to the HD "Cheat Sheet" plate (page 90) to build your meals, especially when out at a restaurant.
- Remember: When eating an HD-friendly food, add high-hydro foods. For example, pair a yogurt snack (HD-friendly protein) with high-hydro fruits or veggies.
- Do not go for more than 4 hours without eating. When you go for long periods without the proper nutrients, your body instinctively goes into starvation mode and your metabolism slows down. All calories consumed thereafter will be stored as fat, and you don't want that!
- Think whole foods, not processed!
- Start meals with a limitless salad or soup.
- Move your body!
- When you feel like you are about to make a bad decision, take a breath. Close your eyes and picture your end goal. You can do this!
- Eat mindfully and live decisively.

12 WEEKS OF DECISIONS

Here I am introducing Maya the Busy Mama again. During her 12-week weight-loss journey, a number of important issues were revealed. While your journey will unfold differently, you may relate to some of Maya's triumphs and trepidations as well as the decisions she focused on. The HD plan is a 12-week commitment; as such, it's common to start strong and lose some stamina toward the middle and end.

So think of the below almost like a dialogue you'd hear as a fly on the wall in my office. The back-and-forth between Maya's frustrations and my recommendations are a peek into the feelings behind those weekly weight check-ins and how you can stay encouraged.

WEEK 1: 147.2 pounds

I never have time to concentrate on myself, and it has gotten out of control. I need you to tell me what to do!

Decide today to make the time. Skipping breakfast is not an option. Use quick and easy recipes, like While-You-Sleep Chia Oatmeal or Microwave Chia Egg Soufflé. Remember to shop and have the ingredients on hand.

WEEK 2: 142 pounds

I cannot believe I lost 5.2 pounds! I felt so much better this past week. I shopped and prepared and felt in control. But I am nervous because I have several birthday parties for the kids and a dinner out with friends this week.

Decide not to go out to a party hungry. Instead, eat a piece of fruit or a handful of nuts beforehand so you are at a 5 or 6 on the hunger scale. Don't sabotage your hard work. You are doing it!

WEEK 3: 142.4 pounds

I am so frustrated! I can't believe I gained almost half a pound. The only bad thing I did was have one and a half glasses of wine at dinner. Otherwise I stayed strong!

Decide to stay encouraged. It is not unusual to have a big loss and then a week where nothing moves. You introduced alcohol—which is on the IF list—prematurely. However, your body was detoxing and responding, so go back to your attitude from the first week. There will be time to introduce IFs again.

WEEK 4: 139.6 pounds

I haven't been in the 130s in years! I stayed strong this past week, and it paid off. I wasn't ready to introduce IF foods after the first week. This feels so good!

Decide to start incorporating exercise into your journey. You are making time for yourself now, and it is reflected in your weight-loss results and how you feel. You understand the effects of having control over your food patterns and what you put in your body. It's time to move now.

WEEK 5: 136 pounds

I was so scared to weigh in because I had some IF foods. I needed that drink on Friday night! I even had a bite of my son's frozen yogurt. But I have been exercising and doing all the other steps on the HD plan!

Decide to keep logging! Your logs revealed that you can have an IF food during the week and still get incredible results. That's encouraging! Your exercise routine and your mindful HD eating are what got you results this past week.

WEEK 6: 136 pounds

I am relieved my weight stayed the same. I thought I would have gained for sure. I was in many situations where it was easy to make bad decisions. I tried to eat fruit, instead of desserts, at every social event. I definitely lost some control this past week.

Decide to regroup and pay attention to portion sizes this week. You can overdo it on good foods, like fruit, too. In place of a fruit snack, grab a free HD snack option, like the Nori Vegetable Wrap or Vegetable-Chia Miso Soup.

WEEK 7: 133.4 pounds

I really got back on track this week. I am still not where I want to be, but I feel like I can get to the 120s soon! I also feel like I need more grab-and-go snack choices, especially since I am traveling this week with the kids and afraid I'll make bad decisions.

Decide to look over the list of grab-and-go bars and snack ideas for your travels. You have not tried bars yet as a snack; they could help you in these instances as a quick option.

WEEK 8: 131 pounds

I never in my life thought I could travel and lose weight. I was so nervous about it!! The kids have their foods and I now have mine.

Decide to acknowledge the progress you have made. You were not even in your own environment and you stayed focused. You were properly prepared for your trip mentally and physically. You paid attention to what you put in your body and it paid off.

WEEK 9: 131.6 pounds

I am aggravated! I want to get into the 120s and I am still trying. I haven't been perfect, but I have changed so many bad habits.

Decide not to detach from your HD journey. You must reward yourself for the changes you have made while being realistic about your outcome. Last week you really went out a lot and had IFs on several occasions. A 0.6-pound gain makes sense!

WEEK 10: 130.4 pounds

Last week scared me so I started to pay more attention to the decisions I was making when I dined out. I also added a day of exercise because I wanted to see a '2' after that '1'!

Decide to always be mindful when dining out. You can be social in HD- you just need to ask for your meals prepared properly and be aware of you portions. Remember the HD "Cheat Sheet" plate. Ask for what you want—be a diva!

WEEK 11: 130.6 pounds

I don't think I am meant to be in the 120s. I feel stuck.

Decide to stop backsliding. Review your previous "decisions" and figure out where you need to honor them. You are living in HD. You just have to pull in the reins because you are not at your goal yet.

WEEK 12: 124.8 pounds

I decided to eliminate all IFs—no alcohol or desserts—and restart strong. It paid off. I feel like I completely understand how to live in HD. My goal of 120 will be accomplished!

Decide to keep deciding. Are you where you want to be? This isn't a sprint. This is a new lifestyle. You will get to 120, and with all you have learned on this journey, you will stay there.

HD FREEBIES

Everyone loves foods that "you don't have to think about." Having some go-to foods that are guilt free is really nice for when you are feeling low on energy, experiencing a sudden dip in the Hunger Determination Scale, or just want to occupy your tastebuds. I have already emphasized that high-hydro vegetables are limitless on the HD plan, so it will come as no surprise that many of these freebies are, well, vegetable oriented. However, there are a couple of sweet surprises as well.

HIGH-HYDRO OPTIONS

HD Crudité (page 165)

Broccoli Soup (page 193)

Good Decisions Soup (page 195)

Vegetable-Chia Miso Soup (page 198)

Nori Vegetable Wrap (page 227)

Any steamed high-hydro vegetable

Gazpacho Soup (page 194)

SWEET TOOTH OPTIONS

Vanilla Agar Pudding (page 220)

Chocolate Mousse Agar Pudding (page 220)

Lemon Custard Agar Pudding (page 220)

Free Frozen Fruit Skewer (page 222)

CRUNCHY SNACK OPTIONS

Kale Chips (page 226)

Roasted Chia Nori Strips (page 229)

HYDRO-BOOSTING SWEET TREATS

Good Decisions Vanilla Chia Pudding (page 222)

Good Decisions Cacao Chia Pudding (page 222)

STEVE, 54,
Lost 45 Pounds

Before HD: I just knew I needed to get healthier. And I was ready to take control of my health for the long term.

Starting strong: When I first met with Keren, she gave me her famous plate demonstration. She arranged plastic foods on a plate so that vegetables were on one half and a lean protein and a carb were on the other and said, "This is what I would like two of your meals to be a day." Then she took away the carb and said, "This is what I want one of your meals a day to look like." I liked this because I'm a busy guy, and I needed someone to just give me a set plan to follow. I also make sure to exercise 5 days a week—3 days in the gym, 2 days of golf.

Unexpected bonus: I've always been the guy who goes full tilt with everything, but this is a very balanced way of living and eating. You feel better about yourself, physically and mentally.

Lesson learned: Addition by subtraction. This means HD swaps, like sweet potatoes for white potatoes or ordering a salad with salmon at lunch instead of a burger. But it's what I'm not eating—like no cheese, watching avocado, limiting intake of carbs, having dressing on the side—that makes the difference.

Sustaining in HD: Anything in life that you want to be successful at, you have to plan for—including living in HD. For instance, if I have an early morning meeting, I now know that I need to plan what I'm going to eat beforehand so I don't end up grabbing something bad or that won't keep me full. I've done more food shopping with this regimen than I've done since . . . I honestly can't remember. And I don't find it a hassle at all.

Inspiring words: Following the HD plan is painless. It's a truly sustainable and sensible way to eat.

7

STILL FOCUSED AND ADDING IFS

"If you are interested in something, you will focus on it, and if you focus attention on anything, it is likely that you will become interested in it. Many of the things we find interesting are not so by nature, but because we took the trouble of paying attention to them."

—MIHALY CSIKSZENTMIHALYI

Some of my most highly motivated clients stick to the principles of Start Strong—the core of the HD plan—until they reach their goal weight. But if you're like most, or if you have a lot of weight to lose, you'll likely have a taste of your pre-HD life before you reach your goal. Let me say here that, as a nutritionist, sure there are foods I wish you'd steer clear of forever. There's a lot of junk out there that really has no business being put into people's mouths and bodies. But I am also a realist. I too get cravings for unhealthy foods. So I teach my clients that these foods aren't "bad." Just *IF*-y.

That is to say, they are infrequent foods (IFs): the foods and drinks that aren't great for our health or maintaining a stable weight. But let's face it, unless you live in a bubble or on a vegan, raw-foodie commune, you'll be facing them often throughout your HD life. So learn to think:

IF I eat this food, I know it is not the best for me.

IF I eat this food, I will be very mindful of its placement in my diet and make sure it does not contribute more than 200 calories at a time.

IF I eat this food, I will thoroughly appreciate the experience, slowly and sensually, being mindful of every bite.

IFs include cheese, cake, and fried foods, just to name a few—and, as you might have guessed, I don't advocate consuming any of these foods on a regular basis. Here's the full IF list.

- Alcohol
- Artificial sweeteners
- Butter and margarine
- Canned foods with added salt or sugar
- Dairy foods (cow's milk, cream, ice cream)
- Cheese (gets its own category)
- Fried foods
- Processed foods with added sugar or salt
- Red meat or processed meat (like bacon, ham, sausage)
- Refined sweets (like cakes, candy, cookies, pastries, pies)
- Salt
- Snack foods (chips, pretzels, basically anything in a bag)
- White pasta and white bread

And one more . . .

- Pizza (another big IF)

Now I can't tell you how many times I've had a client look over this list, laugh, and then say in a very serious manner, "What? There must be nothing to eat on your plan!" Well, after reading through Chapters 5 and 6, you know that's untrue. The HD plan food lists are extensive. Many of us are simply used to eating a number of these IFs on a daily basis. And that is no way to live in HD. But you are not a robot, and foods on the IF list are not out of your life forever. On your HD journey, you just have to view these IFs differently.

That's what the Still Focused in HD phase is all about. You begin by incorporating one IF per week with great mindfulness. All of the other Start Strong guidelines apply. You are still using tools like daily food logging, weekly goal setting, and weekly weight checks. And you are becoming more in tune with your body. How do you know you're keeping on track? A pivotal living-in-HD moment is when you have indulged in an IF food and still feel in control and healthy and your waist is getting smaller.

One note of caution here: Before you can succeed in Still Focused, you need to be honest about the kind of person you are because some of us are "ALL or NOTHINGS." This is a phrase my clients and I came up with for individuals who struggle with the concept of *slowly* adding IFs to their routines. These people claim that if they have just one bowl of ice cream, one brownie, or a handful of potato chips, the floodgates will open, all bets will be off, their jaws will become unhinged, and they will be back to living fuzzy.

If you can relate to this phenomenon, please pace yourself throughout the Still Focused phase. A big part of living in HD is understanding what works best for *you*. There is a moment in everyone's journey where being mindful of certain foods starts to get easier. The desire to "shove in" the bad stuff goes away. It doesn't always happen at the 14-day mark. Sometimes it takes longer. But it *does* eventually happen.

Now I want to explain why the foods mentioned earlier made the IF list. I hope these explanations will help you see that I am not just trying to torture you or take away all your fun. (Don't forget: It's also pleasurable to buy a new, slimmer clothing size; to sleep better; or to just have more energy during the day!)

ALCOHOL

Before I started my practice, I had no idea how many of you revere your alcohol! It happens to be first because the list is in alphabetical order, not because I want to be a party pooper right from the start. I'm not preaching that you can never relax after a stressful workweek or dealing with your screaming kids with a nice, big glass of wine or a margarita. In fact, many times you will see me out doing just that. I like to have a drink at the end of a hectic week, too! But if you are trying to lose weight, or drinking has turned into a nightly routine, you may need to rethink your alcohol habits.

Alcohol is toxic. And this is evident when the toilet bowl becomes your best friend after one too many drinks. Unfortunately, many of us

You get drunk when the liver, unable to keep up with your drinking, can't get to the excess alcohol and start processing it. The alcohol circulates in your body until the liver is ready. That's when you start to feel inebriated, with slurred speech and crazy behavior.

can relate to that scenario. (Not if you are reading this and are under 21, of course!) Your body does not recognize alcohol, so it is metabolized differently than other foods and drinks you ingest. After you gulp it down, it is absorbed quickly into your bloodstream, and the liver starts its work metabolizing the toxins. Unfortunately, while your liver is busy concentrating on this job, your body can't properly process the carbs, protein, and fat you also ingested, so the food your liver couldn't get to is stored on your hips!

I emphasize this scenario for those of you who feel like having 100 to 200 calories of an alcoholic beverage per night is no big deal. "What's 200 calories? It's not breaking the calorie bank," some of you might say. The trouble is, all calories are not created equal. When you are first learning to live in HD, I want your metabolism to be unspoiled. Alcohol works against your metabolism—no matter how few calories of it you ingest. Of course, alcohol lowers your inhibitions as well, which causes you to reach for the cheese fries when you otherwise would refrain! If you're not convinced that alcohol needs to be on the IF list, consider this: Alcohol is a diuretic, so it causes water depletion, which causes you to lose important minerals, such as magnesium, potassium, calcium, and zinc, all of which you need to help maintain fluid balance and strong muscles.

As to the "What should I drink?" question, here are my answers. Skip the cosmopolitan or vodka with orange juice. All sugary mixed drinks are no-nos. Spirits have fewer carbs. Think gin or vodka and seltzer with a twist of lime or lemon. Beer or wine is an option, too, but that doesn't mean you can drink the entire bottle of wine or chug one beer after the next. Nurse your one drink and enjoy.

The bottom line: Take all this information under advisement. If you are desperately trying to lose pounds, it is a good idea to avoid alcohol for a while to help get your metabolism back on track. There will be room for an occasional drink eventually.

IF you have an alcoholic beverage, drink water too. In fact, alternate sips to avoid that dehydrated slump many people get when they drink.

IF you drink alcohol more than twice a week, give your liver a break. Let it metabolize food, not alcohol!

IF you have a drink, nurse it and enjoy it. You'll appreciate it more when it's not an everyday indulgence.

ARTIFICIAL SWEETENERS

As the owner of a sweet tooth myself, I can understand the allure of artificial sweeteners. Sweet cravings satisfied with no additional calories? Sound too good to be true? It is.

I'm talking here about the:

Yellow packets (Splenda, sucralose)

Pink packets (Sweet'N Low, saccharin)

Blue packets (Equal, aspartame)

These sweeteners may have no calories, but they *will* make you unhealthy and fat. When I first started working as a nutritionist, I preached this to clients because I wanted to promote natural foods. I had read the studies and thought it sounded "on trend" for my field. But, admittedly, I didn't have the conviction for the subject that I do today. Now I honestly, wholeheartedly believe (to my very core) that artificial sweeteners will not keep pounds off. I have seen this proven time and again.

I have had clients whose diets consisted of many of these sweeteners. (Remember Vivienne, the Plump Know-It-All, from Chapter 3?) Yet when they removed these sweeteners from their diets, the pounds came off. Why? These products work by stimulating sugar receptors without causing a rise in blood glucose levels, like sugar does. But they have been shown to trigger massive cravings for sweets, which can sabotage weight-loss efforts.[1]

There have been many studies linking a sweet taste, whether delivered by sugar or artificial sweeteners, with increased appetite. One study clearly demonstrated that aspartame also increased subjective hunger ratings compared to glucose or water.[2] In another study, aspartame, acesulfame potassium, and saccharin were all associated with heightened motivation to eat more items selected on a food preference list.[3]

Remember, your body *still* needs to metabolize these fake sweets. Do you recall how hard your body works to metabolize alcohol? These sweeteners were concocted in a laboratory, and our bodies have to work hard to metabolize anything foreign and unnatural. Artificial sweeteners certainly fall into this category. If you use a sweetener, switch to stevia.

BUTTER AND MARGARINE

The difference between butter and margarine still confuses people. I completely understand! We hear so many different morsels of advice from the media about what to eat and what not to eat, and these two spreads have gotten a lot of airtime. To better understand why butter and margarine are on the IF list, here's a quick overview of saturated fat and trans fat.

Saturated fats are derived mostly from animal products, though some, like those found in palm kernel oil and coconut oil, are plant based. These fats, which are solid at room temperature, have been shown to raise serum (total) cholesterol and LDL (bad) cholesterol levels. Butter is guilty of all of the above: It is made from cow's milk, is solid at room temperature, and has a lot of saturated fat—7 grams per tablespoon, in fact. The limit on saturated fat is 10 grams per day. That's a lot of fat for a little smear! I have had clients explain their butter obsession to me, and their portions typically well exceed the limit. Not to mention that a single tablespoon of butter also contains 102 calories.

IF you are a butter fanatic, stay mindful, especially when cooking. It is harder to control portions when cooking, and the fat calories add up fast.

IF you choose butter as a spread, limit your portions. One tablespoon will still give you the creamy kick you crave.

IF you are used to eating a lot of cookies and cakes, remember that these treats contain not only sugar but also fat from butter!

Trans fat is mostly man-made. It is created by adding hydrogen to vegetable oils through a process called hydrogenation (or partial hydrogenation), which gives these oils a longer shelf life. Trans fats were once touted as a great invention: The theory was that foods (like muffins, for example) made with trans fats instead of animal-based saturated fats would now be heart healthy because they contained no cholesterol. (Only animal products contain cholesterol.)

Here's the kicker, though: Trans fats, like saturated fats, increase blood cholesterol levels and the risk of heart disease. They tend to raise LDL cholesterol—while also lowering HDL (good) cholesterol—when eaten in quantity. Also, trans fats can make our blood platelets stickier, and that's just gross.

This information was eventually acknowledged in 2006, and an FDA ruling on labels encouraged food manufacturers to reduce or eliminate trans fats from their products. However, many packaged foods will advertise "No Trans Fats," even though they contain some; manufacturers are allowed to make this claim if there is 0.5 gram or less of trans fat per serving. Ideally, we should be limiting our trans fat intake to no more than 1 gram a day, so 2 servings of a "0 trans fat" product could still put you at the daily maximum!

How can you avoid trans fats? Look for hydrogenated oil or partially hydrogenated oil in ingredient lists. I know it seems ludicrous that you have to do detective work, but that's why the ingredients are listed.

IF you want the butter flavor, my advice is to go for the real thing. Margarine spreads and "diet" butters are man-made, which can wreak havoc on your metabolism.

IF you must have that nonbutter spread, please read the labels. Natural products, like Earth Balance's Buttery Spread (which is vegan), are a good alternative.

DAIRY FOODS

Many of my clients think dairy foods are on the list because of lactose, a sugar found in milk. Lactose intolerance is a common enough term that even those who don't suffer from bloating, diarrhea, or constipation after consuming dairy know a bit about the condition. (Someone who is lactose intolerant lacks the enzyme to properly break down the lactose in dairy products.)

Lactose is a legitimate concern for some people, but there's another reason why I recommend eating dairy with caution. Dairy also contains casein, a protein that is hard for the body to digest. If you have a tough time with casein, your body can display symptoms that include eczema, nausea, bloating, dizziness, and exhaustion. Of course, many dairy products are also high in saturated fat and, if we're talking ice cream, high in sugar.

We want to give our digestive systems a break on the HD plan. I have had many clients discover that they feel a lot better when they consume dairy with caution or eliminate it from their diets altogether. And there are so many delicious alternatives on the market now. I use unsweetened almond milk on cereal and in puddings and smoothies. I love almond milk! It's creamy and refreshing, plus it contains no sugar (assuming you're buying the unsweetened varieties; vanilla-flavored almond milk has some sugar in it). Not to mention, it's a good source of calcium, too.

By the way, much of this cautionary advice applies to fat-free milk products as well. Fat-free milk still contains casein and sugars. Cheese, however, deserves its own heading.

IF you want a dairy kick, use unsweetened almond milk.

IF you have a dairy product, pay attention to the way you feel afterward.

CHEESE

Cheese gets its own section because it is beloved by so many. In fact, the mere thought of temporarily eliminating cheese seems to cause as much distress as the prospect of cutting out alcohol for many of my clients. Why is cheese IF-y? It's high in fat, high in calories, and pretty much the opposite of hydrophilic (it has zero fiber). And, as mentioned in the previous section, some people are generally intolerant of dairy. But if you're a cheese *mangia*-er, you should probably cut out cheese altogether on the core HD plan.

Cheese has more casein than any other natural source. This is because of the way cheese is made. The curds are mostly composed of casein, so it's hard to digest. On a more practical note, cheese can be sneaky. It's easy to put away 4 ounces without batting an eye. Reduced-fat or nonfat "cheese foods" are even worse on our systems, given the tons of extra ingredients that are added to make them cheese-ish. Many clients find that eliminating cheese has a really positive impact on their bodies and their health. Even my Gouda-loving clients feel better equipped to put cheese in its rightful IF place when they eliminate it for a time.

When you're ready to handle cheese as an IF, consider beginning with cheeses made from sheep's or goat's milk. These are easier on your digestive system. Aged cheeses like Parmesan are also easier to digest. Parmesan is actually a great choice because it packs a ton of satisfying flavor in a small amount: Just a 0.5-ounce portion of the real stuff sprinkled on salads or in soups brings a lot of cheese flavor.

IF you choose cheese, please be hyperaware of portions. An ounce of really good cheese (about the size of two dice) can satisfy your craving.

IF you choose cheese, combine it with a high-hydro fruit or vegetable.

IF you're in a place where cheese and crackers are being offered before your meal, remember that the calories add up quick.

FRIED FOODS

French fries, fried chicken, doughnuts, onion rings, mozzarella sticks, tater tots, egg rolls, fried shrimp, funnel cakes—oh my! I don't think this category comes as much of a surprise. You will not lose weight or maintain a healthy body if you regularly eat fried foods. Fried foods are

HD FOOD CALCIUM AMOUNTS

Many of my clients are concerned they won't get enough calcium if they cut dairy from their daily diets. But so many foods on the HD plan are *great* sources of calcium. Check out this list.

- Almond milk
- Beet greens
- Bok choy
- Clams
- Collard greens
- Cowpeas
- Crabmeat
- Dandelion greens
- Fortified cereals (various)
- Kale
- Oatmeal
- Ocean perch
- Okra
- Rainbow trout
- Salmon, wild
- Sardines
- Soybeans
- Spinach
- Tempeh
- Tofu
- Turnip greens
- White beans

immersed in hot oil, and they're often doused in fatty batter as well.

Fried delicacies are usually consumed outside of the house—at restaurants, street fairs, fast-food joints. (I mean, not many of my clients are whipping out the deep fryers at home.) I mention this because these eateries are most likely using hydrogenated oil, lard, or palm oil to fry these foods in. These are "bad" fats, and you're better off avoiding them.

IF you are going to eat fried foods, do so rarely and watch your amounts! A couple of onion rings are a reasonable IF indulgence. The whole basket is overkill.

IF you regularly crave fried fare, experiment with healthy baked versions at home. For example, there's a recipe for Sweet Potato Fries on page 204 and one for Parsnip Fries on page 202.

PROCESSED FOODS

Check this out:

INGREDIENTS: ENRICHED BLEACHED WHEAT FLOUR [FLOUR, FERROUS FULFATE, "B" VITAMINS (NIACIN, THIAMINE MONONITRATE (B1), RIBOFLAVIN (B2), FOLIC ACID)], SUGAR, CORN SYRUP, WATER, HIGH FRUCTOSE CORN SYRUP, PARTIALLY HYDROGENATED VEGETABLE SHORTENING (CONTAINS ONE OR MORE OF: SOYBEAN, CANOLA OR PALM OIL), DEXTROSE, WHOLE EGGS. CONTAINS 2% OR LESS OF: MODIFIED CORNSTARCH, CELLULOSE GUM, WHEY LEAVENINGS (SODIUM ACID PYROPHOSPHATE, BAKING SODA, MONOCALCIUM PHOSPHATE) SALT, CORNSTARCH, CORN FLOUR, CORN DEXTRINS, MONO AND DIGLYCERIDES, POLYSORBATE 60, SOY LECITHIN, NATURAL AND ARTIFICIAL FLAVORS, SOY PROTEIN ISOLATE, SODIUM STEAROYL LACTYLATE, SODIUM AND CALCIUM CASEINATE, CALCIUM SULFATE, SORBIC ACID (TO RETAIN FRESHNESS), COLOR ADD (YELLOW 5, RED 40). MAY CONTAIN PEANUTS OR TRACES OF PEANUTS.

The food industry allows many, many, many different food additives. And the fact that many of these additives are deemed safe does not mean it's a great idea to eat them. Artificial flavors, sodium nitrite, color dyes, preservatives—these should not be part of an HD life.

IF you get a headache from constantly reading your food labels, take an aspirin and reach for an HD snack.

IF you must reach for food made in a factory (for me, it would be

Twizzlers), follow the HD guidelines and appreciate that it's an occasional treat.

RED MEAT AND PROCESSED MEAT

Many carnivorous clients give me a dirty look at this point. There is so much conflicting information on whether meat is good or bad for you. And trust me, many clients achieve success on the HD plan after reincorporating their beloved meat. I am not saying that red meat needs to be off the table forever, but here's the bottom line: Red meat is hard to digest. Meat is mainly protein-dense animal muscle, and it's high in saturated fat.

Red meat can also up your chances of getting heart disease. When Harvard researchers tracked the food choices of 37,698 adult men and 83,644 adult women for up to 28 years, they found that eating 3 ounces of red meat (about the size of a deck of cards) every day increased one's chances of dying during the course of the study by 13 percent.[4]

What are the dangers? Well, it's that saturated fat. The iron in red meat, which in excess can be bad on the heart, is also a problem for some. And certain carcinogens can be formed during the cooking of meat as well.

It is important to eliminate red meat during the Start Strong phase because your metabolism could really use the break. If you are a regular meat eater, this may force you to look at other protein options, like fish, lean chicken, or, my HD favorite, beans.

But IF eating meat is your **IF** choice:

1. **Choose your cut wisely.** Round, sirloin, or tenderloin (including New York strip and filet mignon) have about the same amount of fat as a skinless chicken breast. Avoid prime and T-bone.
2. **Spring the extra $ for grass-fed beef, if you can find it.** It has higher levels of omega-3 fatty acids than grain-fed beef does.
3. **Remember the HD "Cheat Sheet" plate from Chapter 6.** Portion rules apply! Many of us eat meat out at restaurants, and, unfortunately, restaurants overportion *a lot*. Share your entrée or take half of it home for your dog.

Processed meat is just that—a meat that has been through chemical or salt processes to extend its shelf life. Sausage, hot dogs, bacon, and many luncheon meats fall into this category. There are usually very high levels of sodium in these products. The sodium count can be up to three times more than you would consume if you were eating a sandwich filled with fresh meats. That's no way to live in HD! All this sodium not only leads to bloat but also can be hard on the heart.

Processed meats also often contain nitrates (not to mention higher calories and fat). Diabetes experts say that nitrates lessen your secretion of insulin and have negative effects on the body's glucose levels. Harvard researchers recently did a study that showed that eating just one serving a day of processed meats was linked to a 29 percent risk for diabetes. One serving, for example, is just two slices of salami or a hot dog.[5]

IF you want a deli sandwich, it is best to use fresh meat.

IF you do buy packaged meats, always read ingredient labels. Do not purchase if made with sodium nitrite or monosodium glutamate.

REFINED SWEETS

Here is another "no duh" IF group. There are no diet plans (that I know of) that say it's okay to stuff your face with candy, cake, cookies, doughnuts, and sugar-sweetened juice. When it comes to weight loss, pretty much all of us know that refined sugar products are on the no-no list. Yet our nation is *obsessed* with sugar. If we ever want to solve our obesity epidemic, our excessive sugar intake has got to stop. But you don't have to mourn your fudge brownies forever. And you can still enjoy your movie nights on the sofa, munching on Twizzlers. You just have to learn to keep sugar in its place.

This is difficult for so many people though. Some clients were sent to me by their doctors after blood tests revealed prediabetes and the potential for a slew of other health problems. I even had a client who desperately wanted to conceive a child and couldn't because of her weight. The doctor told her that she had to lose weight and change the way she ate before they could start to tackle her fertility concerns.

Addressing bad sugar habits was a doctor's order for these individuals, and they still found it difficult to accept that they even had a problem. They were addicted. Why is this? Marcia Pelchat, PhD, a food psychologist at Philadelphia's Monell Chemical Senses Center, explains it well: "We're born to like sugar." Even infants show an early preference for sugar. Way back when, a taste for sweetness may have led our ancestors to prefer ripe fruits and skip the bitter—and poisonous—ones. Not to mention, sugar can ease pain; it has a natural analgesic effect.

Whether people can become physically dependent on sugar is still being debated in scientific circles. Some animal studies suggest that it's quite possible. Researchers have noticed the brains of animals given sugar have the same changes in dopamine levels as that of drug addicts. Yikes! All I know is that people who indulge in refined-sugar treats every day have a hard time quitting. But to live in HD you *must*, at least in the beginning of your journey. You just have to quit cold turkey.

> Stevia rebaudiana Bertoni is a plant native to Paraguay. This green-leaved sweetener is noncaloric, natural, and safe to cook with. And it has medicinal properties to boot. Stevia leaves are estimated to be 150 to 300 times sweeter than refined sugar.

Mind you, I am talking about refined white sugar here. Natural sugars from high-hydro fruits are still okay. And there are many sweet-tooth fixes available on the HD plan to help get you through cravings. In the end, you won't crave the white stuff like you did in the past. This will be a big step in your HD journey, so just give it a chance.

IF you need a sweet boost, high-hydro fruits are a great option.

IF fruit won't cut it, try stevia. Stevia can regulate blood glucose levels and impede those sugar cravings. I use it in oatmeal, shakes, and in the HD freebie desserts, like the Vanilla Agar Pudding or the Good Decisions Cacao Chia Pudding (pages 220 and 221, respectively).

IF stevia is not to your taste, try honey or natural maple syrup. (Kids love maple syrup.) But remember, although natural, these options are caloric and affect blood sugar levels, so use them mindfully.

SALT

We all need some salt in our diets to help our bodies maintain fluid balance and transmit nerve impulses. Plus, our muscles rely on it to contract and extend (i.e., move properly). The problem is that many of us eat too much salt—way too much salt. Dietary guidelines recommend limiting sodium intake to less than 2,300 milligrams a day. (If you are 51 or older; are African American; or have high blood pressure, diabetes, or chronic kidney disease, it's recommended you stop at 1,500 milligrams a day.) However, the average American consumes more than twice that.

The culprits? Processed foods, frozen dinners, and a lot of restaurant meals are all major offenders. And then there are those of us who salt everything out of habit, even foods that already have salt on them.

How is excess salt harmful to health? Sodium attracts and holds water, leading to increased blood volume, which makes our hearts work harder, which leads to high blood pressure. When we live in HD, we want to avoid overworking our hearts.

There is also water retention to consider. Many of my clients complain of water retention. Do you feel like your rings are cutting off your circulation after eating Japanese food? Do your ankles look like cankles after a family barbecue? Then you are probably sensitive to sodium, and all that salt is interfering with your flat-belly aspirations.

Unfortunately, taste alone may not tell you which foods to avoid. A bagel may not taste salty, but a typical 4-inch oat bran bagel contains about 600 milligrams of sodium. And a slice of whole wheat bread has around 100 milligrams. The nutrition facts label found on most packaged foods can help you navigate this landscape. Those labels also list whether the ingredients include salt or sodium-containing compounds, such as:

WANT TO CUT BACK ON SALT?

Eat fresh. Most fresh fruits and vegetables are naturally low in sodium. Fresh meat is lower in sodium than cold cuts or anything processed. Look for fresh meat that hasn't been injected with a sodium-containing solution. Check the label or ask your butcher.

Go for reduced-sodium varieties. If you do buy processed foods, or boxes of grains (like rice) with added seasonings, choose those labeled as low in sodium.

Watch out for salt that's not in a saltshaker. Sodium gets into our systems from all kinds of condiments. Soy sauce, many salad dressings, dips, ketchup, mustard, and relish all contain salt.

Try lemon juice. The juice and grated peel from citrus fruits can spice up your meals (as can herbs and spices).

And remember: Just because the recipe calls for salt, doesn't mean you have to add it, or at least not in the full amount.

- Baking powder
- Baking soda (also called sodium bicarbonate)
- Disodium phosphate
- Monosodium glutamate (MSG)
- Sodium alginate
- Sodium citrate
- Sodium nitrite

1 teaspoon of salt = 2,400 milligrams of sodium
1 tablespoon of soy sauce = 1,000 milligrams of sodium

Your taste for salt is acquired, so you can learn to enjoy less. Try to avoid anything with more than 400 milligrams per serving. Decrease your use of salt gradually and your tastebuds will adjust. Some foods will even start to taste *too* salty. Your preference for the salty stuff will diminish, allowing you to enjoy the true taste of the foods you eat.

IF you use salt, don't shake unconsciously. One shake equals around 150 milligrams. It can add up quickly.

IF you need to spruce up a bland dish, try kelp powder (my favorite) or experiment with different types of herbs. You will discover flavors you didn't know existed.

SNACK FOODS—CHIPS, PRETZELS, OR ANYTHING IN A BAG

In Chapter 5, snack foods like chips were listed in the HD-friendly category if they had fewer than 100 calories and at least 3 grams of fiber per serving. So I had to include this food category on the "IF" list because that is one hard rule to abide by!

Many bagged snack items are high in calories, high in fat, deficient in fiber, and oh so difficult to portion. Usually just 10 chips will get you 100 calories. (Have you ever tried to eat only 10 potato chips? Not only is it difficult, it's not terribly satisfying either.) And the same goes for all of the bagged snacks lining the shelves of Whole Foods or Trader Joe's. It's easy to get seduced by the newest potato, soy, bean, or tortilla chip that promises "all natural" ingredients. But I don't need to remind you that "all natural" does not mean "diet." These foods can quickly sabotage your HD effort.

If you are looking for a crunch, try the Kale Chips (page 226), Roasted Chickpeas (page 231), HD Popcorn (page 229), or Roasted Chia Nori Strips (page 229).

If you choose to eat snacks from a bag, do buy high-fiber varieties.

WHITE PASTA AND WHITE BREAD—BASICALLY, ANYTHING MADE FROM WHITE FLOUR

Refined white flour has been stripped of wheat's most nutritious parts. Which is to say, white flour might as well be sugar. The stripping process means that white flour–based foods are instantly absorbed upon reaching the intestine. Unlike the fiber-rich, high-hydro carbohydrates that take much longer to be digested, absorbed, and broken down into energy, white flour immediately raises your blood sugar levels.

After you eat white flour, your body has two choices: burn it off immediately or store it as fat. If you eat a lot of white flour products and do not burn them off with exercise immediately (and who among us jumps from bread basket to treadmill?), they will mainly be stored as fat. This is not good for your body, for sure, but I implore you to stay away from white flour mainly because it leaves you hungry! The instant elevation of your blood sugar and the eventual crash leaves you tired and—worst of all for your HD journey—ravenous.

Also consider the nutrients that get lost in the refining process.

- About 50 percent of the unsaturated fatty acids
- Almost 100 percent of the vitamin E
- 50 percent of the calcium
- 70 percent of the phosphorus
- 80 percent of the iron
- 98 percent of the magnesium
- 50 to 80 percent of the B vitamins
- And many more nutrients (there are simply too many to list)

IF you want a carbohydrate fix, stick to the HD food lists. There is a definite place for pasta in your HD life, but in the beginning of your journey, ½ cup of a grain like barley is more satisfying than ½ cup of pasta.

IF pasta is your vice, choose healthy varieties like whole grain, buckwheat, barley meal, oat bran, brown rice, or bean.

PIZZA

I can't have an IF food list that doesn't mention pizza. It's quick, easy, and—let's admit it—pretty delectable. It's often the standard food at children's birthday parties, football gatherings, and lazy-night dinners. But its allure is precisely why it has to be on the IF list. Pizza is high in calories, high in fat, hard to digest (all that cheese!), and void of hydrophilic fiber. Often when you eat a slice of pizza, you are hunting for something else to eat soon afterward. That is why it should be an infrequent indulgence.

Yet it is the one food you will most likely have a confrontation with on your HD journey. A common scenario is a child's birthday party. I can't tell you how many times a client has told me they were at a Gymboree party and *had* to have the pizza because there were no other options: "What was I to do? I had no choice but to have a slice, or two."

Gotta tell you: This is a situation that should never develop when you are committed to living in HD. You need to plan ahead. When you're headed to a party where pizza will probably be the only food option, don't go hungry. This is especially true if you are in these predicaments a lot, which is the case for many of us with young children. Pizza can be enjoyed occasionally. You just need to put it in its place.

IF you want a pizza fix, make it yourself on an HD-friendly carbohydrate, topped with ¼ cup of sauce, lots of high-hydro veggies, and (after Start Strong) 1 tablespoon of Parmesan.

IF you find yourself at a pizza joint, order a slice with tons of high-hydro vegetables and no cheese. It's good. Really.

IF you want the real thing, indulge infrequently.

After following the Still Focused in HD strategies for a while, you will become much pickier about what IFs you indulge in. You might even painlessly drop some of your IFs altogether, only keeping ones you truly love. Me? I stuck with black-and-white cookies, Twizzlers, and that occasional glass of wine.

What's *your* IF? What foods do you imagine you could never live without? If you decide to only *infrequently* eat your favorites, forgoing the IFs you don't really love won't be so difficult.

RANDI, 54,
Lost 18 Pounds

Before HD: I was going through some tough family stuff and using nighttime binging to make myself feel better. Only it didn't make me feel better. I would consume massive quantities of calories—salty carbs, sugars, and fats—late in the evening. It was causing tremendous depression and weight gain.

Initial goal: Lose 20 pounds and stay off statins.

Starting strong: It's amazing how Keren's words inspired me to make the decision to take control of my weight and my health. I knew I was doing the wrong things, and the extra weight was depressing me even more. The Start Strong phase really felt incredible. I felt like a new person after 2 days on the HD plan. I am so excited to continue what I am doing; I already lost 10 pounds!

New foods: Greek yogurt with chia seeds and berries. Decision Nutrition Chia Chips. Nori wraps. Club soda with a drop of cranberry juice plus a lemon or lime wedge.

Unexpected bonus: When you stop the late-night eating, you're hungry when you wake up, as normal people should be, but I didn't know that! Now I eat breakfast and look forward to it, which I had never done before.

Lesson learned: If I don't take care of myself, I can't be of any help to others. So I have to be at peak performance, whatever that might be.

New mantra: I start the week prepared with foods that are healthy to eat and will make me feel better.

Sustaining in HD: My husband and I make soup on Sunday and look forward to planning meals for the week. We cook at home a lot more. Plus, I can really taste my food now. For instance, I don't put sugar in certain foods anymore, just a bit of cinnamon or a little vanilla. On the HD plan, your tastebuds open up and your whole palate changes.

What's next: I would hope restaurants catch up on preparing healthy dishes that aren't tasteless and boring and upping their HD vegetable portion sizes. They are definitely getting better but have a ways to go.

Inspiring words: I eat very mindfully and I do *feed* myself. I wake up and I'm not in a bad mood or anxious or depressed. I can get up earlier *and* I can stay up later at night (because I'm not putting myself in a sugar coma). I'm coming at things in more thoughtful, less reactive ways. I even remember things more. I'm more confident with my work, with my family, with everything! I have a new lease on life.

By the end of 12 weeks, Randi lost 18 pounds of her 20-pound goal. Her weight loss slowed down after the Start Strong phase, but she remained consistent and slowly achieved 91 percent of her end goal. She has kept the weight off and still remains mindful of how her emotions affect her eating decisions.

P3

LIVING IN HD

8

HEALTHY HD ALTERATIONS

"Stay committed to your decisions, but stay flexible in your approach."
—TONY ROBBINS

Over the years, I've had many new clients express concerns about being able to adhere to my plan because of a food allergy or intolerance, health issue, or personal lifestyle choice made for ethical, religious, even political reasons. If you are ready to start living in high definition, let me reassure you the HD plan is highly adaptable. Often my main concern is working through *why* a client wants to eliminate a particular food group from their diet.

The number of people with food allergies who walk into my office has definitely grown since I began my practice. According to a study by the Centers for Disease Control and Prevention, food allergies among children increased approximately 50 percent between 1997 and 2011. It's hard to admit I have been in the nutrition field for that long but, yes, it is true, and that is a staggering jump.

Scientists have many theories as to why this is happening. Some think it's simply that we are reporting allergies more often, while others trace it to excessive cleanliness. (The hygiene hypothesis maintains that the antibacterial product craze interrupts the normal development of immune systems.) Regardless, food allergies are a real concern.

I need to stress, however, that a food allergy is not the same as a food intolerance. The avoidance of certain foods has become very in vogue lately, and it's important to understand the differences.

Food intolerances can be truly uncomfortable. My middle son has a gluten intolerance, and I can attest to how difficult it was to watch him squirm in pain. He went through every test in the book. Every condition that would classify him as having a wheat allergy—for instance, a rash in response to a skin test—was ruled out, yet he still hurled over with stomach cramps after eating a bagel. So we decided as a family to eliminate gluten from his diet. (Gluten, for those who haven't encountered it already, is a protein found in wheat, barley, and rye.)

There are many reasons why someone might be sensitive to a particular food. The most common reasons are lack of the enzyme needed to fully digest the food (as with lactose intolerance) or irritable bowel syndrome, which is a chronic condition that causes constipation, diarrhea, and intestinal cramping.

A true food allergy causes an immune system reaction that affects numerous organs in the body. In some cases, an allergic reaction to a certain food can be life threatening. People allergic to peanuts or tree nuts know what I'm talking about. Severe food allergies are scary and serious, and in these cases ingesting even a tiny amount of the allergen can immediately bring on anaphylaxis, in which the throat swells and blood pressure drops to dangerously low levels.

In contrast, food intolerance symptoms are generally less serious and are typically limited to digestive problems, hence my son's bagel distress. The symptoms usually come on gradually and don't involve an immune system reaction. Digestive issues may include nausea, vomiting, cramping, and diarrhea. Other symptoms could be a tingling mouth; hives; or swelling of the lips, face, tongue, or throat.

If you have a food intolerance, you may be able to eat small amounts of the offending food without trouble. My son, for example, seems to be able to eat some sauces and candies that contain gluten, but bread products never agree with him. You may also be able to help prevent a reaction by taking certain measures. For example, if you have lactose intolerance, you could drink lactose-free milk or take lactase enzyme pills (such as Lactaid) that aid digestion.

Celiac disease has some features of a true food allergy but isn't one. It's an autoimmune disorder triggered by eating gluten. If you have celiac disease, eating gluten triggers an immune response in your small intestine, and over time, this reaction causes inflammation that damages the small intestine's lining and prevents the absorption of some nutrients.

Other diet limitations, like the decision to avoid animal products, are personal lifestyle choices. Which, of course, does not mean the reasons for the choice aren't serious.

Let me assure you that if your avoidance of a certain food is a personal choice, the HD plan can be adjusted. If it is due to a food allergy or intolerance, it is adjustable as well. If you suspect you are having an adverse reaction to a particular food, my best advice is to visit a doctor to find out whether it's due to a food sensitivity, allergy, or celiac disease, just so you understand the true consequences of consuming that food.

HD FOR THE GLUTEN FREE

The gluten-free phenomenon needs to come first on this list. Many clients want to eliminate gluten from their diets for no other reason than having read that some celebrity, like Kim Kardashian, is on a gluten-free plan (so why wouldn't it work for them, too?). How well it might work, though, really depends on the approach.

Gluten-free products line the shelves of our supermarkets today much like fat-free products inundated supermarkets in the 1980s. Everyone then thought that if they ate fat-free foods, they would lose weight and be healthy. I thought this too! I loved my SnackWell's cookies, especially because I believed I was eating a "free" food with every delicious bite. But as time went on, I became more ingredient-savvy and began to understand that if fat is removed from a food that typically has it, other ingredients must be added to make up some of the taste and mouth-feel difference. In the case of my cherished cookies, it was sugar.

Does the same hold true for many gluten-free products? Of course! I am telling you this because I have dealt with so many clients who fell prey to the gluten-free allure. They thought they would lose weight like a postpregnancy Heidi Klum if they filled their carts with all of these gluten-free foodstuffs. They ate gluten-free breads, pastas, cookies, and bars, trusting that these foods were the answer to their well-being. Sound familiar? These products, however, do not equal weight loss or health.

When people truly are gluten intolerant, have celiac disease, or simply want to see how eliminating gluten from their diets will make them feel, I can support this. The guidelines for the HD plan still stand, just with a few easy modifications. As far as all the gluten-free cookies available, they are not "diet" or "free," but, hey, gluten-free people deserve their IFs too!

The HD plan is easily adjusted to a gluten-free lifestyle because it stresses whole eating. This is important because the fresher the food, the more likely it is to be gluten free. By the same token, the more processed the food, the higher the odds that it contains gluten. Many deli meats contain gluten, for example. And processed foods belong in the IF category.

When you cook at home, it is easier to keep track of what's in your meal. So if you are sensitive to gluten, bring on those aprons. Make your own HD soup instead of buying soup at Whole Foods; it's easy, healthier, and often cheaper.

All high-hydro vegetables, high-hydro fruits, high-hydro proteins, HD-friendly proteins, and hydro-boosting chia seeds are allowed when going gluten free on the HD plan. Barley, rye, farro, and, in some instances, oats would be eliminated from the high-hydro carbohydrate list. (It just depends on the individual's sensitivity to gluten.)

For high-hydro carbs, the focus would be on amaranth, buckwheat, brown rice, quinoa, acorn squash, butternut squash, parsnips, and sweet potatoes (any potato is free of gluten, but I love those sweet potatoes). As far as HD-friendly cereals and breads go, become a label reader. If you are craving that bread or cereal kick as *one* of your carbs, I modified the rules for you a bit: Look for products that are

Oats were deemed "unsafe" for gluten-sensitive people largely because of cross-contamination issues. Oats were often grown next to wheat and barley in fields, then processed, milled, and even transported with these other grains. Somewhere along the line, some of the gluten from the wheat and barley would "wear off" on the oats. Today, more and more growers are dedicating fields and equipment to oats alone, so it's less of a problem.

gluten free with 150 calories or less per serving, 2 grams of fiber or more, and 6 grams of sugar or less.

Beware of condiments. Gluten can be hidden in mustards, soy sauce, and other types of sauces, so again, please read labels. Tamari and Bragg Liquid Aminos are wheat free.

HD FOR THE DAIRY FREE

I already discussed that cutting out dairy during the Start Strong phase allows your digestive system to take a break from hard-to-digest casein. Almond milk is used as a replacement for cow's milk, and cheese and ice cream are eliminated (except as IFs in later phases), so avoiding dairy is already part of the HD plan.

Start Strong principles do allow for a Greek yogurt because lactose-intolerant and milk-sensitive individuals can do well with this type of yogurt as a protein option.

If you live completely dairy free because of diet restrictions or beliefs, eliminate yogurt from the HD-friendly protein list. There are many dairy-free yogurts available in supermarkets today, but please be aware of the sugars added to many of these products. Try to avoid any that contain more than 7 grams of sugar per 6-ounce serving.

HD FOR THE NUT FREE

A nut allergy is a serious issue. Whether you are specifically allergic to peanuts or tree nuts, many people who deal with this affliction choose to avoid *all* nuts. I've had many clients who have children with a peanut allergy, and they do not want anything containing nuts in their homes. I completely understand.

In this case, you would eliminate all nuts and nut butters from the MUFA list in the HD plan guidelines. Avocados and olives can remain. You would also replace almond milk with another dairy-free option, like soy, rice, or coconut milk. (Please buy unsweetened varieties!)

Some people are sensitive to coconut, so ask your doctor about consuming coconut products if you have a tree nut allergy.

HD FOR THE VEGETARIAN/VEGAN

People interpret their lifestyle preferences in all kinds of ways. Some people call themselves vegetarians because they eat no animal flesh but still eat eggs, dairy, and fish (sometimes called pescatarians). Then there are lacto-ovo vegetarians, who eat no fish and no animal flesh but say yes to eggs and dairy. Then there are vegans, who do not eat meat of any kind and also no eggs, dairy products, or processed foods containing these or other animal-derived ingredients, such as gelatin.

Regardless of your preference, you still have to live in HD. I add this because there are plenty of vegetarians and vegans with unhealthy eating habits walking around. There are vegetarians who don't eat vegetables. (I always love that one.) There are vegetarians who eat only french fries, pasta, and cheese pizza. (Hey, there's no meat in any of those foods, right?) There are vegetarians and vegans who gorge on chips and pretzels. None of these eating habits lead to living in HD.

When vegetarians and vegans walk into my office, desperate to find a way to lose weight and feel more energized, I tell them the HD plan is adaptable to any possible vegetarian variation. Tofu and tempeh are HD-friendly protein options, and there's a long list of high-hydro proteins. The other HD guidelines still apply.

DIABETES AND HIGH CHOLESTEROL

If you are on a diet for diabetes, you need to watch your sugars. And if you are on a low-cholesterol diet, you have to be mindful of your saturated fat intake. Frequently clients come to me with concerns about one or both of these medical matters, and they think that I can come up with some special diet just for them. This is not the case. The HD plan is appropriate for either of these populations. Clients with dangerously out-of-control blood sugar levels have gained control of this problem just by following the HD plan. And I've also had clients with severely elevated cholesterol levels who followed the HD plan and were able to lower their numbers and avoid medication.

THE REST OF THE HD LIFESTYLE

Now I want you to think about puzzles for a moment. One puzzle piece looks like a blob of nothing, but put all the pieces together and a clear, bright image emerges.

This is how you have to look at your overall health and well-being. I have gone over many important pieces so far: (1) making the decision, (2) when to eat, (3) how much to eat, and (4) what to eat (and even what modifications may be necessary). These are all crucial pieces that will help bring your HD life into focus. Here are some additional puzzle pieces you might want to consider.

SUPPLEMENTS

Supplements can truly help improve digestion and increase metabolism. That said, supplements are no magic bullet. No supplement alone will help you lose stubborn pounds. While I think taking a daily multivitamin can benefit everyone, I am also a big believer in changing your diet first. If you really want to improve your weight and health, you must partake in every HD guideline discussed thus far.

I generally won't even discuss supplements with clients until they are in charge of their diets, including eating decisions, eating patterns, and portion sizes. Once they have these things under control, supplements can be an *added* element of the HD way. Of course, some clients aren't interested in taking any kind of supplement and think it's all snake oil.

However, supplements *are* helpful for some. So many clients feel they have a dysfunctional metabolism when they first come to me. And I understand the temptation to blame a slow metabolism if weight management has been a persistent issue. Remember, though, that just fixing your eating patterns (as discussed earlier) can vastly change your metabolism. The following supplements can help, too, once the basic steps have been taken.

B vitamins: Take a B-100 complex daily to help metabolize carbohydrates and proteins.

Coenzyme Q10: Take 100 milligrams daily to stimulate your metabolism.

Kelp: I love those seaweeds! One kelp pill daily can help support your thyroid gland if you feel like you have a sluggish thyroid. That's because kelp is a great source of iodine. If you are already taking thyroid medication, then don't begin kelp supplements.

A healthy digestive system also leads to a healthy metabolism. Many times I see clients who have been living the high life. (Remember Stan the Constant Socializer?) When you have been eating processed foods, drinking lots of alcohol, and filling your plate with portions that could feed a horse, your insides will not be in the best shape. Chia seeds are wonderful for getting your digestive system back on track, as are all the HD guidelines. Here are some supplements that can provide an added boost.

Aloe vera juice: Aloe is a gelatinous, hydrophilic plant. No wonder I like it! If you suffer from digestive issues or want to clear out those toxins, aloe juice can be helpful. Take 1 tablespoon daily as needed. It has a strong taste, so you may want to add some reduced-sodium tomato juice to disguise it.

Digestive enzymes: If you feel like your digestion is failing you, take one capsule with every meal. This can help with nutrient uptake and make you feel more satisfied. I have often suggested digestive enzymes to clients who feel they have *many* food intolerances. A good, consistent regimen of these enzymes can help relieve gastrointestinal discomfort in these instances.

Probiotics: All of us can benefit from taking a daily probiotic supplement to aid digestion.

Triphala: Take it once a day in the evening to clean out your colon. Many times I use this colon cleaner for just 2 weeks to get my digestion back on track after a vacation or stretch of nonoptimal HD eating.

CLEANSES

I don't advocate juice cleanses in my practice. Clients sometimes tell me that they tried one in the past and felt great while doing it. But once regular eating resumed, they felt terrible and every pound lost on the cleanse returned.

Fact is, any weight loss results achieved on juice cleanses are not sustainable. You feel great on cleanses because you're not consuming toxic foods or drinks. No alcohol, no refined sugars, no dairy, no processed foods—the body reacts to this experience positively; it is like a detox. So is the HD plan though, but unlike a cleanse, you chew real food and get all the nutrients you need. It's more realistic, and it's definitely more sustainable.

EXERCISE

You didn't think this could be a healthy diet book without some talk of exercise, did you? Exercise is a very important piece of the HD puzzle. But I always stress the word *piece*. Remember Remy the Chubby Perpetual Exerciser and Evan the Enormous Iron Man? I bring these two up again because I have encountered many people who exercise and do not live in HD. They use exercise as a license to eat.

Once you have learned to manage all the principles of the HD plan, exercise will be an integral piece of the puzzle, bringing your body and mind benefits that you never imagined possible.

If you are already an exerciser, that's fantastic! Keep it up! Or perhaps you have been frustrated because you *do* exercise and *still* have a hard time looking at your butt and paunchy stomach in the mirror. I've heard it all before. Learn (and live) the core principles of the HD plan and keep on pumping!

If exercise is not a part of your daily life, or if you are always making excuses about exercising, here are the reasons why you need to decide today to make exercise a part of your HD life.

Exercise can help get you to your HD weight goal quicker. Exercise burns calories. The more intense it is and the longer you do it, the more calories you burn. And on the HD plan, a consistent exercise regime will absolutely lead to downward movement on the scale. Remy and Evan didn't see this because their eating lifestyles were out of control. Once you apply the HD plan guidelines to your everyday life, exercise will be your ally.

Exercise is crucial to maintaining your HD weight. There will come a point in your HD life when you achieve your desired weight. When you are sustaining in HD, it is natural that those IFs will make appearances more than ever before. This is because you are at your goal weight—looking hot, getting compliments everywhere you go—and the reins will start to loosen. Whether it's a drink, a cookie, or an ice cream cone, these foods can be consumed with much less guilt when you exercise. The problem with Remy and Evan was that they were eating IFs every day—more than once and in large quantities—which is why their exercise routines were failing them. But start to place IFs in your week with mindfulness, and exercise can literally make those foods "free." They will be burned off before they even have a chance to touch your hips.

Exercise reduces your risk for health conditions and disease. Of course we want to take off the pounds and keep them off for good, but we also want to live long enough to enjoy our hot bods. There is no refuting that exercise can help combat and prevent heart disease, high blood pressure, type 2 diabetes, stroke, metabolic syndrome, certain types of cancer, and arthritis. Research has shown that if you are physically active, your HDL (good) cholesterol levels are boosted and triglycerides are decreased. And exercise can help control your blood sugar and decrease your belly fat. Of course we want to look fabulous, but the health benefits of exercise cannot be denied, especially when the food piece has been addressed.

Exercise makes you happier. Regular physical exercise can stimulate brain chemicals that put you in a better mood. Have you ever forced yourself to go to that aerobics class or for a jog, and when you're done, you feel like you can conquer the world? Of course, that feeling is easily forgotten the next time you have a free hour and the choice of running or browsing the Internet for shoes on sale at Saks Fifth Avenue. Or is that just me? But remember, there is no doubt that exercising regularly improves your outlook, which is a very important component of living in HD.

Exercise can increase your resting metabolic rate. When you increase your lean body mass, your body will burn more energy. This is why it is important to incorporate weight training into your exercise repertoire. Doing so can increase your resting metabolic rate by as much as 15 percent, which helps you burn calories even when you are sitting on your butt browsing for shoes on sale on the Internet. That is what gets me to do my squats.

Exercise can improve your sex life. As if all the above was not enough, I thought I'd give you one last motivator. Sexual dysfunction is affected by your health. If you take care of your health—addressing all the important pieces of the puzzle, including exercise—sex can be better than ever. A study at the New England Research Institutes found that regular, vigorous exercise can help lower the risk of impotence. The researchers studied more than 600 middle-age men who reported having no problems with impotence at the start of the study. After 8 years, the men who exercised regularly were less likely to have impotence problems.[1] In addition, a study in the *Journal of the American Medical Association* found that sexual dysfunction is more likely among men with poor physical and emotional health. It also found that sexual dysfunction negatively impacts sexual relationships and overall well-being.[2] And, after all, it only makes sense that your nightly activities will be more fun if you are becoming more svelte and feeling happier and more energized.

There you have it—the many reasons why it is so important to make exercise a part of your HD life. And by the way, the key is *consistency.* You don't have to get all fancy on me. I know there are a million different classes, boot camps, centers, and trainers. (And more power to you if you partake.) But many people think exercise has to be a whole big production and then decide they just don't have the time for it. And as a result, they suffer the consequences. I love my non-fancy workouts. I love running. You can do it whenever you want (no class times). I add on some situps, squats, and dumbbell lifts after my run, and I'm done in under an hour. Trust me, we can all find the time to do the things we really want to do. And this brings me to the very last piece of the HD puzzle.

LYSSA, 53, *Lost 13 Pounds*

Before HD: I was typically a very thin person. And then last year I started to eat randomly. Nothing satisfied me. I'm not even a person who loves food! I was just constantly in the house grabbing things. I had worked with a nutritionist in the past, but her whole setup pushed packaged goods, and I don't eat packaged goods. So there I was picking and noshing, and nothing good was going on (or in).

Starting strong: I liked the HD plan's emphasis on fruits, vegetables, and fresh foods. Also, I stopped using all the bad artificial sweeteners. I use stevia products now, like Truvia, once in a while. Keren said, "Have some oatmeal with chia seeds." And I gagged (for real). "I will never eat oatmeal in a million years," I said. Now I eat oatmeal every day.

Oatmeal was Lyssa's block food! (See page 14.) I encouraged her to give my favorite high-hydro grain a fighting chance. She complied and that was it. Oatmeal was "unblocked," and now she enjoys it every morning. Remember: Be aware of your own block foods and give them a try. You never know!

New foods: Honeycrisp apples. Lemon water. Steamed spinach with grilled salmon. Almonds with an apple.

Never misses: Almond M&M's.

Unexpected bonus: My friends say, "Oh, my God. You're eating all the time." They were so used to seeing people barely eat anything on "starvation" diets.

Lesson learned: I was eating a lot of double proteins; like, I would put chickpeas *and* chicken in my salad. I was subscribing to the adage that eating a lot of protein is fine. With Keren's help, I debunked a lot of the myths I was operating under.

Sustaining in HD: I barely look at restaurant menus because I know that the way many dishes are prepared is not what I want. So I usually say to the server, "I just need a piece of fish steamed with some steamed vegetables." I've noticed that when you're trying to get something accomplished, people appreciate it; they don't give you a hard time. Then when the server brings my plate, I always say, "Thank you so much. This is exactly what I wanted."

Inspiring words: It's more than just a state of mind. My body's not craving all the bad stuff.

9

CURING EXCUSITIS

ex • cus • i • tis
ik-skyüz-īt-əs
noun
1. A condition in which a person makes excuses.
2. When the justification for your actions obscures your path toward living decisively.

You will not find *excusitis* in the dictionary. I made it up. The word came to me after counseling numerous individuals who suffered from this phenomenon at some point during their HD journey. I'll be honest. Not every single one of my clients lives happily ever after in HD, and I think that's harder on me than it is on them. This very last piece of the puzzle—treating excusitis—is critical. If excusitis is not cured, it can sabotage *every* step you take toward a better life.

Excuses cloud your decision-making process. I once worked with a woman I'll call Maggie. She signed up for the HD program and seemed truly motivated. Let's face it, my 12-week, in-person HD program costs a lot more than this book, so you'd think someone who had plunked down cold, hard cash would be ready to roll. And Maggie seemed to Start Strong, losing a few pounds the first week and a couple the next and then nothing the third week (not an unusual occurrence as you adjust to the plan, as discussed in previous chapters). But when she lost nothing the fourth week, I knew something was going on.

We reviewed her weekly decisions, and Maggie finally 'fessed up.

Turns out, she had two work dinners in a row, then she had to work late on a project one whole week and couldn't get to the grocery store, then she got her period and *needed* a major chocolate fix, and then . . . and then . . . and then. . . . It was clear to me that Maggie had caught a *bad* case of excusitis.

Maggie never was able to find the cure, and I couldn't find a way to help her. She left me after 6 weeks at practically the same weight as when she started. To Maggie, all of her excuses were very valid, and she let them consume her. To me, well, they made me kind of sad, honestly.

It happens to everyone: There you are, loving your new eating plan, and nothing can touch you, until you hit a few days in a row—or a week—where nothing goes as planned. You get off track. Or you *do everything right* and still the scale doesn't budge. At this point, it's tempting to use your fender bender/busted boiler/menstrual cycle to justify pigging out or, worse, quitting altogether. You start thinking about how hard staying focused is and how nothing is happening for you anyway, so you might as well have (a couple of) homemade brownies at the PTA meeting or the (stale) Danish at the marketing meeting (after all, the discussion went long and you were famished). And you start to make *excuses, excuses, excuses.*

Nearly every one of my clients "catches" excusitis sometime during the 12-week HD program. I've been plagued by it myself. As a working mom with three kids, I can assure you it's not difficult to come up with legitimate reasons for why I don't have time to get to the supermarket to stock up on healthy foods: *I want to go home and take a shower, and I need to get my bare dirty nails done.* Or why, while at the supermarket, I absolutely needed to buy that black-and-white cookie to spike my energy: *I had the hardest day; the teacher called to tell me my kid was acting up, and all my clients complained about their weeks to me.* Or why, on my way to buy a rotisserie chicken and broccoli, carrots, green beans, and brown rice for sides, I stopped at the pizza place instead: *Steaming veggies and boiling water for the rice seems like a lot to do when I get home, and the kids won't eat it anyway. I want to hang with my husband and boys, not stand by the stove and clean; I am pooped!*

But like a bad cold can turn into pneumonia, a minor case of excusitis can escalate. Let too many days go by without treating it, and excusitis will seriously threaten your weight-loss efforts.

There is no known vaccine, but I can offer some relief from whatever symptoms you might be suffering from during your HD journey, and it starts with awareness. Be aware of the excuses entering your mind and sabotaging your forward momentum. Because they will! Believe me. The best we can do is remain aware of our self-sabotaging mantras and be armed with ways to squash them.

Below you will find the most common excuses I have heard over the years (if I listed them all, this would be a 200-page chapter!) and some successful treatments that got clients back on the path to living in HD.

I am too stressed/exhausted with my kids/studies/job to go shopping for/cook healthy foods. There just aren't enough hours in the day.

In the Stone Age, when we were hunting for our meals or gathering berries to feed ourselves and our families, lack of time might have been an issue. In the 21st century, there's an app for that. At the very least, smartphones and the Internet are your friends. A great many (if not all) areas of the country offer grocery delivery services, which let you order your HD fixings online and have them delivered. (If you work long hours, have your groceries delivered to the office and then bring them home.) Also, most supermarkets offer a variety of precut vegetables, which helps make prepping for meals a snap. If you really want someone else's cooking, there are plenty of healthy options. Many Asian restaurants offer a "health menu" full of steamed vegetables plus tofu, shrimp, or chicken.

I could go on. The HD plan stresses planning menus, meals, and snacks for the upcoming week and shopping accordingly. By following the suggestions above—plus using technology and being willing to pay delivery fees—your excusitis will be alleviated.

It's my birthday month/the holidays/my vacation/ a sales conference.

I want you to take out your calendar right now and look through it. I promise you, you will have "something" every month, whether it's a birthday, party, work event, or holiday. You don't live in a hydrophilic-vegetable bubble and you never will. So you have to learn to apply the HD principles throughout the events that are part of everyday life. When you find the HD formula that works for you, it will all come into focus and your excusitis will quickly clear up.

I got my period. My hormones made me eat everything in sight!

Surprise! Surprise! I hear this a lot from my clients (just the female ones, of course), and I say, "Seriously? Getting your period is news?" You know it's going to come every month, so you shouldn't be blindsided by hormonal cravings. Like everything else, if you have a plan for your premenstrual meals and snacks, you can get through those days without screwing up your weight-loss progress. Whether it's finding an HD sweet treat or having your IFs mindfully at this time, you can figure this one out. Coming down with a severe case of excusitis every month is unacceptable!

My mother/husband/friend brings me foods that I shouldn't eat.

I hear this complaint often. Change is hard, and sometimes even a change for the better is hard on people we love and who love us. Sadly, *you* living your life in HD might be threatening to the status quo, and that can be scary for some of the people around you. If this is the case with you and your loved ones, assume your potential HD saboteur means well; after all, we're probably talking about mothers who associate nurturing with food, husbands who are used to being providers, and friends who treasure you in part because you're their reliable rom-com-DVD-and-pint-of-Cherry-Garcia buddy. Give your pork rind–bearing loved one the benefit of the doubt. Not eating what this person puts in front of you probably isn't going to make-or-break the relationship. The bottom line: No matter what's put in front of you, the *decision* to eat it or not eat it—or to eat just one or two bites of it—is *yours* and yours alone.

I need my chocolate/wine/dessert every day.

Got a daunting food weakness? Join the club! But if you find that you hit the vending machine every time you experience an energy lull at work, you're seriously undermining your progress to an HD life. Decide to cut your consumption of these foods back to once a week as an IF treat once you're past the Start Strong phase. Find an HD substitute for the rest of the week. For chocolate, try the Good Decisions Cacao Chia Pudding (page 221), Chia Cacao Yogurt (page 219), or Chocolate Mousse Agar Pudding (page 220). Theresa the On-the-Go Gobbler didn't think she could live without her nightly two glasses of pinot noir, but by making wine her twice-weekly IF, she found it a whole lot more enjoyable than when she was guzzling mindlessly. Once you gain control over the foods you think you need, you will see the pounds drop, and there is nothing like a slimmer waistline to help cure excusitis.

I find exercise boring.

Okay. Then find a way to make exercise un-boring because you need to get your blood pumping for your health, body, and mind. If you hate the treadmill, join a class that's more fun. If you can't stick to a schedule, there are so many online workout videos or DVDs you can use on your own time. Stop thinking of exercise as a chore you need to do, and start thinking of it as time for yourself amid a crazy, hectic day. When you exercise, you can "go to another place." Listen to music while you dance, run, stretch, walk, box, lift, take the stairs—just *move*. My point is, exercise can become as addictive as any bad-for-you habit. Once you realize how much you enjoy exercise, you won't want to make excuses any longer.

I just had a baby.

Having a baby changes your entire world. Your body is no longer just yours while that little life is nurturing itself in your womb. It's a miracle, and at times it really sucks. I have done it three times, and each time I feel like I rented my body out for a good 18 months to my very own miniature extraterrestrial. It's a process that you have no choice but to give in to. And yes, I do have those psycho mamas who come in 4 weeks after their babies are born and want to know why they aren't back to their prebaby bods. Please, ladies, give yourselves a break! Do not look at magazines and gawk at Gisele Bundchen's flat new-mom stomach and sink into a depression. You don't know what her struggles were, and it doesn't concern you anyway. Please allow adequate time after giving birth before you start obsessing over your prebaby figure. However, I have seen how the stresses of a new baby can take over a mom's ability to make good food decisions long, long, long after the baby is thriving and hardly a baby anymore. In this case, you need to stop with the "baby" excuses. Sure, life is more challenging—you have a whole other human being to consider at all times!—but your body will respond to the principles of the HD plan, and being a healthy, hot mama is so much sexier than succumbing to excusitis.

It's not really me; it's just impossible to lose weight as you get older.

I hear this again and again. A fortysomething will explain to me that her old diet trick of eating one meal a day isn't working any longer or that refusing all carbs just isn't translating into a size 4, but when she was younger, this was a cinch! Well, here are the facts. Research has shown that most people's metabolisms decrease by 0.5 percent per year after the age of 25. The three main physiological factors that slow down a person's metabolism are a decrease in muscle mass, a change in hormone levels, and a decrease in the caloric needs of internal organs. This is why your old bag of tricks does not work any longer. However, all three of these factors can be controlled by lifestyle changes. You need to focus on changing your eating patterns so your metabolism runs efficiently. You need to increase your lean body mass by exercising in order to increase your resting metabolic rate. And you need to change the *types* of foods you eat. Get a new bag and fill it up with these new tricks, and, before you know it, your metabolism will rev up like a twentysomething's. No more excuses.

My kids come first–I'm very selfless–and I need to tend to their needs before I tend to my own.

I get it. I really do. If you are a parent, you have a lot on your plate. There have been times when I have literally forgotten about my own needs because I was so focused on my children's happiness and well-being. And who has the time? How much can we do? We are psychiatrists, cooks, maids, playmates, workers, drivers—the list goes on. But our children need us, and they need us happy. Whenever I am in one of my self-righteous modes, my mother reminds me to put my own oxygen mask on first and then attend to my children. Happy parent = happy child. Remember this the next time your excusitis flares up.

Healthy foods cost too much.

A bag of chips or a Big Mac costs less than a pound of Brussels sprouts or a bag of apples. It really can be infuriating that eating healthy seems to cost more. And why is this? The more processed the food, the longer it lasts, and therefore the cheaper it is to sell. Fresh foods deteriorate fast, so they cost more. I really do empathize. I have had to decrease our spending before and was shocked when I realized such a hefty portion of the monthly budget was spent at the market. (My Internet shopping episodes did less damage!) But I don't want food costs to stop you from living your life in HD. I had to make the decision to stop my Internet shopping episodes until things got better for us. I prioritized, and you might need to as well. And there are other ways to make it easier on your wallet; you just have to make the decision to do these things. There are definitely markets where you can find amazing deals on healthy produce. You would comb the Internet for the cheapest car that still provides the features you need, and you can do the same comparison-shopping with healthy food. You can also make shopping lists so you are prepared when you arrive at the market, which always saves money. Educate yourself on what fruits and vegetables are in season, therefore cheaper. It is possible to follow the HD plan on a budget. It's a very important decision to make, so you have to get over the excusitis because you're worth it and deserve to live in HD.

The freshman 15 is inevitable.

New environment. Away from mom and dad. Crazy hours. Drinking (when you turn 21, of course!). It's a challenge for this group to keep up healthy eating patterns, but the freshman 15 is not a natural rule of the universe. School campuses offer so many healthy options now. I make sure that my young adult clients understand the importance of the hunger scale and eating patterns. I encourage them to be equipped with HD snacks during their classes so they don't make bad decisions when they get to the cafeteria. I also stress that late-night eating can truly sabotage their goals of not packing on the pounds. If you stay up studying all night, be ready with high-hydro vegetables and high-hydro fruits to fill you up. Scarfing down a bag of chips nightly will always result in the numbers on the scale going up. So I beg you, college boys and girls, please get a hold of your excusitis because no one can get away with these erratic eating behaviors, not even the young.

I am going through menopause.

I cannot stress enough that menopause doesn't mean accepting being fat as your fate. It is just not true. As explained earlier, your body does change as you get older, and this happens to everyone. But you can fight the pounds with the principles of the HD plan. I have had countless menopausal women discover their HD formulas and sustain their ideal weights. I beg, beg, beg you: Don't let menopause be the reason you fall prey to the "old lady" mind-set. In this case, *do* look to celebrities for inspiration. Check out Michelle Pfeiffer, Christie Brinkley, Katie Couric, Jaclyn Smith, Susan Sarandon, Meryl Streep, Jane Seymour, Sharon Stone, Sophia Loren, Jane Fonda, Helen Mirren, Diane Sawyer—all over 50 and smoking! Right? No more menopause excusitis.

I want a busy social life, so it's impossible to watch what I eat with any real consistency.

I know that it's often tough to order in a big group or say no at the family table. But sometimes, it's okay to be a bit of a diva (or divo, for the men). Think Beyoncé, J. Lo, Tom Cruise, and now you! I have had to remind so many clients that it's okay to ask for what you want when you are working so hard toward a tough goal. When you are living in HD, you are bound to encounter all sorts of situations that may derail your progress. In these instances, just ask for what you want. It may mean asking how an entrée is prepared or scouring the supermarket for a hard-to-find product. (Supermarkets actually have staff members. If you can't locate something, ask somebody! Chances are they'll appreciate a friendly interaction with a customer.) If you ask, you get. This is especially true if you are polite and sweet about it. And most importantly, don't be ashamed of your healthy HD alterations. I can't tell you how many times clients have professed that they were embarrassed to request a diet modification, like swapping 500-calorie, oil-laden veggies for 60 calories of steamed ones or asking for a sauce on the side. This pertains to both men and women who want to lose weight, reclaim their health, *and* eat out a lot. Your friends and family will have to understand that you are changing the way you approach your health and diet. And who knows? You may have a positive influence on someone you care about who's in the same predicament. What you have been doing thus far has not worked. Make your healthy changes and be proud. Excusitis crushed.

It was in front of me, so I had to eat it.

Remember the 226 food decisions we are faced with in a day? Well, sometimes a tempting dish will be placed right in front of you while you're on your HD journey, and then you may have to "kill the beast." My strongest diet memory is being in the college cafeteria with my best friend who would "kill" our food daily with salt, ketchup, and mustard so we wouldn't take another bite once we were satiated. We would get the dessert of the day, every day, take a bite, and then chant, "Kill it! Kill it!" We were always pleased with our disgusting heap of mixed condiments and our self-control. Truth be told, I am still friends with her and recently witnessed the murder of a fudge brownie at a mutual girlfriend's birthday dinner. Part of living in HD is about making the decision to stop before you're overfull and finding the self-control to do so (even if you have to resort to stupid tricks). You don't have to be as violent about it as we were, though. But then again, to cure your excusitis for good, maybe sometimes you'll have to be.

My best friend/mother/sister/father/brother does whatever she/he wants and looks great. It's not fair that I can't do the same.

This is the last example of excusitis I will give you. I end on this one because I hear it all the time, and it's the one that bothers me the most. I know I mentioned some celebrities as inspiring examples earlier. And I did this to encourage you, not make you feel inadequate. Remember: Everyone is on a unique journey. No two people reading this book will have the same experience. We are all different. I have three boys; they are all different. I have so many beautiful friends; they are all different. You are you. This is your opportunity. This is your journey to living in HD, and it is yours and yours alone.

LIANA, 25,
Lost 20 Pounds

Before HD: My diet was horrible for a year and a half. I have a gluten allergy and a dairy allergy, so I was buying anything gluten free. And I was eating a lot of meal-replacement bars. Even fruits and vegetables were bothering me. So when I went to see Keren, I brought a list of foods I wasn't eating, and her response to some of the foods on my list was, "You can't eat this? There's no gluten in this!" While this was true, when I did eat these things, I had so much pain and stomach cramping. I was self-diagnosing and my weight kept going up.

I want to take this opportunity to mention the "bar dilemma." Liana dealt with it, and it's a subject that should be addressed. Liana was relying on meal-replacement bars too much as well as focusing on the wrong bars. If it had a gluten-free label, she felt safe and devoured several per day. There are countless unhealthy bars on the market, so it can get very confusing. The right bars—low in sugar, high in fiber—can be eaten on your HD journey *after* you get the hang of the core principles (usually once you've reached the Soaring in HD phase). Then, add them to your grab-and-go collection. My favorites: Kind bars (varieties with 5 grams of sugar or less, counted as an HD-friendly MUFA) and Gnu Foods FiberLove bars (counted as an HD-friendly carbohydrate).

Initial goal: Just to get to the point where I was healthy and happy and felt like myself.

Starting strong: Each week I introduced a new vegetable or fruit in small portions. Slowly, I started eating more of it and got to the point where I wasn't thinking about the fact that I was eating a fruit or vegetable, whereas a couple months before, I was scared to even look at some of these foods because I didn't want to feel pain!

New foods: Kale salad. Cinnamon chicken. Lentil soup.

Unexpected bonus: I lost weight! All I wanted was to be able to eat normal foods. The weight came off when I wasn't even focusing on the pounds—just my health. Also, grocery shopping is a lot of fun now. And the HD plan has me making more meals at home, so I'm saving money!

Lesson learned: You have to stay consistent with the food logging. Once it became part of my routine, it was easier.

Sustaining in HD: Whenever I'm craving cookies or chocolate, I now make agar pudding. The HD plan has helped me find alternatives so I can stay away from things that aren't gluten free or dairy free. I'm not the type to cook, but Keren's recipes are so simple to follow, and I like that a lot.

Inspiring words: I'm living a completely different life now. I will never go back to the way I was eating before.

Through the HD plan, Liana learned so much about how foods *really* affect your body. We added in supplements that can help get digestion and metabolism back on track. In the process, Liana lost 10 pounds *without even trying* because she was finally eating the right types of foods and in the correct patterns.

10

MEAL PREP IN **HD**

Now that you are ready to start living your life in HD, here are some suggestions to get you started in the kitchen.

MAKING CHIA GEL

I always have Chia Gel stored in my refrigerator in a mason jar. This is because of its uncanny ability to increase the surface area of food before your very eyes! There are many recipes in Chapter 11 that use Chia Gel for its consistency and hydro-boosting power. I love adding it to peanut butter, almond butter, hummus, soups, and yogurt.

This is a great HD "hydro-stretch" trick; you feel like you're eating more, but you're actually consuming fewer calories.

Don't forget that you can sneak this gel into your kids' meals for their own hydro-boost. Seeds are safe for kids 6 months and older.

CHIA GEL

2 cups warm water (see note)

⅓ cup chia seeds

In a mason jar, add the water and chia seeds. Cover securely with the lid and shake for 20 seconds. Let sit for 1 to 2 minutes and shake again. The gel is made!

Note the date somewhere on the jar (use a marker on a piece of masking tape if you have to). Keep in the fridge for up to 2 weeks.

Note: Slightly warmed water will form a gel faster.

Not only are you getting a nutritional boost, but you're also displacing calories.

For example:

2 tablespoons natural peanut butter = 180 calories and 16 grams of fat

1 tablespoon natural peanut butter + 1 tablespoon Chia Gel = 110 calories and 9.5 grams of fat

(Remember that 1 tablespoon of raw seeds = 3 tablespoons of gel.)

COOKING HIGH-HYDRO GRAINS

The following chart provides the basic guidelines for cooking high-hydro grains. I refer to these guidelines constantly even though I have been teaching them to others for a while now. (It gets confusing!) Refer to the HD "Cheat Sheet" (page 90) meals and incorporate the grains you feel like having with your meal.

You can also make any of these grains ahead of time and store in airtight containers for up to 5 days. And there are now frozen cooked brown rice packs in the freezer section, which I love to keep handy. But if you want to cook your grains, follow the chart.

	GRAIN AMOUNT (IN CUPS)	WATER AMOUNT (IN CUPS)	COOKING TIME (MINUTES)
Amaranth	1	3	30
Barley, pearl	1	3	40–50
Brown rice	1	2	40–45
Buckwheat	1	2	20
Farro	1	2	25

	GRAIN AMOUNT (IN CUPS)	WATER AMOUNT (IN CUPS)	COOKING TIME (MINUTES)
Oats, steel-cut	1	2	20
Oats, rolled (my preference)	1	2	10–15
Quinoa	1	2	20
Rye berries	1	2	50

HIGH-HYDRO PROTEIN (BEANS)

I definitely recommend keeping prepared beans on hand for a quick high-hydro protein fix. It's so easy, and so many good canned bean options have no sodium whatsoever.

However, there is nothing like whipping up a batch of beans from the dry varieties. The truth is, any time a food is cooked from its natural state, it tastes better.

Personally, I mix it up. When I can, I love to cook dried beans because they're au naturel and cheaper than the already prepared options. The kicker? The time it takes. This is why I lay out some basic bean guidelines for you here.

2 cups dried beans = 1 pound

1 pound dried beans = 6 cups cooked beans

1 cup dried beans = 3 cups cooked beans

½ cup dried beans = one 15-ounce can

1½ cups cooked beans, drained = one 15-ounce can

COOKING DRIED BEANS

1. Discard any dried beans that are shriveled and discolored, and remove any rocks or debris that may be present.
2. With the exception of black-eyed peas and lentils, dried beans require a good soak so they rehydrate for cooking (ahhhh, those beans love their water). In a large pot, cover the beans with water. Place in the refrigerator for 8 hours or overnight.
3. You can also do a hot soak: In a large pot, bring water to a boil. Add the dried beans and return to a boil. Remove from the heat, cover tightly, and set aside at room temperature for 3 hours.

4. Drain the beans.
5. Pour them into the same pot and cover with water again.
6. Place the lid on the pot and bring to a boil.
7. To make beans "gas free," there are a couple tricks of the trade. Kombu has gas-reducing properties that work when added to the beans while they cook. A 2-inch kombu strip should be plenty. Alternatively, you can boil dried beans for 2–3 minutes, cover, and set aside overnight. Discard this water, which contains 75 to 90 percent of the indigestible sugars that cause gas, and cook with freshwater.
8. Reduce the heat and simmer, stirring occasionally, until the beans are tender. The amount of time this takes will depend on the type of bean that you're cooking. Add salt only after the beans are fully cooked. Adding it sooner could prevent the beans from becoming tender.

COOKING TIMES

If you like the ease of canned beans, cook up a large batch of dried beans, divide them into pint-size freezer jars, and stick them in your freezer. They'll be ready to go whenever you need a quick meal.

Adzuki beans—1 hour

Baby lima beans—1 hour

Black beans—1 to 1½ hours

Black-eyed peas—30 minutes to 1 hour

Chickpeas—1 to 1½ hours

Great Northern beans—45 to 60 minutes

Kidney beans (light or dark)—1½ to 2 hours

Large lima beans (also called butter beans)—1 to 1½ hours

Lentils—30 minutes to 1 hour

Mung beans—1 hour

Navy beans—1½ to 2 hours

Pink beans—1 hour

Pinto beans—1½ to 2 hours

CREATING THE ULTIMATE HD SALAD

I am a big believer of incorporating a beautiful salad into your day before your lunch, as your lunch, before your dinner, as your dinner, or as a snack anytime. This probably comes as no surprise since "I'll just have a salad" is seen as the epitome of dieter-speak. The problem, however, is that salads can go terribly wrong in two ways.

1. Additions like nuts (too many), cheeses, fatty and overportioned proteins, dried fruits (too many), and dressings can give your large salad a calorie count equal to that of a bacon double cheeseburger. That's roughly 1,200 calories worth of "diet food" in one sitting.
2. Many times salads are built improperly and don't keep us HD satiated. A common "diet" salad order may be iceberg or romaine lettuce, cucumber, tomato, and some carrots with grilled chicken breast and lemon. While this salad won't pack on the pounds, it won't keep you full for very long either.

So it's time to learn how to build an Ultimate HD Salad. The ground rules are:

- Use ½ cup each of 6 or more high-hydro vegetables, at least, if a salad is your full meal.
- Use ½ cup each of 3 high-hydro vegetables if eaten before your main meal or as a snack.

I love steamed Brussels sprouts or broccoli in mine, but load up on the vegetables that most appeal to you—steamed (if desired), chopped, and ready to add to your base. The more high-hydro veggies, the better.

None of the vegetables listed below will look that surprising to any educated diet-book reader. The focus here is on *quantities*.

DECIDE ON YOUR BASE

The items with an (*) count as a high-hydro vegetable.

Arugula

Bibb lettuce

Boston lettuce

Cabbage (green, savoy, red, napa)*

Collard greens (best slightly steamed)*

Dandelion greens*

Endive

Hearts of palm

Iceberg lettuce
Kale*
Mustard greens (best slightly steamed)*
Radicchio
Red bell pepper
Romaine lettuce
Seaweed
Spinach*
Swiss chard*

These bases are not always available at your nearest salad bar. (If not, hunt down a suggestion card and ask for them!) A great rule of thumb is to make sure half your base is high-hydro (e.g., ½ cup romaine, ½ cup kale). If there is only romaine lettuce available, don't panic. Just pile 6 high-hydro veggies on top.

DECIDE ON HIGH-HYDRO ADD-INS

Choose 5 if your base is high-hydro, 6 otherwise.

Artichoke hearts (but watch out for high-fat marinades)
Asparagus
Bean sprouts
Beets
Broccoli
Broccoli rabe
Brussels sprouts
Carrots
Green beans
Jicama
Kohlrabi
Okra
Onions
Snow peas
Turnips
Yellow squash
Zucchini

Once you've picked from the list above, be liberal with the following HD-friendly vegetables if you desire!

Cauliflower
Celery
Cucumber
Eggplant
Mushrooms
Tomatoes
Water Chestnuts

If you decide to use your 1 serving of an HD-friendly MUFA on this salad, make sure to add the appropriate portion (for example, 15 almonds, ¼ cup sunflower seeds, or ¼ avocado).

And unless you are in the Still Focused in HD or Soaring in HD phases, where you can add 1 or 2 IFS a week, the Ultimate HD Salad means no cheeses, croutons, crunchy noodles, or bacon bits.

Don't forget, adding the appropriate serving size of HD-friendly or high-hydro protein to your salad can make for a terrific meal (for example, 4 ounces of grilled chicken for women and 6 ounces for men)—either as a lunch or dinner.

THE ULTIMATE HD SALAD WITH INTERNATIONAL FLAIR

The following are suggested ways to build salads with an international flavor.

ULTIMATE HD SALAD WITH ITALIAN FLAIR

Arugula/endive mix

Beets

Broccoli

Carrots

Hearts of palm

Onion

Red bell pepper

Zucchini

High-hydro fruit option: 3 figs

High-hydro protein option: 1 cup rinsed and drained kidney beans or white beans

HD-friendly protein option: Chicken or crabmeat (4 ounces for women, 6 ounces for men)

Herb option: Basil

Red wine vinegar (unlimited condiment)

ULTIMATE HD SALAD WITH GREEK FLAIR

Artichoke hearts

Asparagus heads, blanched

Broccoli heads, blanched

Cucumber

Grape tomatoes

Green beans

Onions

Radicchio/romaine mix

Red bell pepper

High-hydro protein option: 1 cup rinsed and drained chickpeas

HD-friendly protein option: Chicken or shrimp (4 ounces for women, 6 ounces for men)

Herb option: Oregano

Lemon-Oregano Dressing (page 190)

ULTIMATE HD SALAD WITH ASIAN FLAIR

Kale

Bean sprouts

Cabbage, shredded

Carrots, shredded

Seaweed

Snow peas

Zucchini, shredded

High-hydro fruit option: 1 medium orange

HD-friendly protein option: Tofu or scallops (4 ounces for women, 6 ounces for men)

Allium option: Scallions

Miso Dressing (page 191)

ULTIMATE HD SALAD WITH LATIN FLAIR

Spinach

Green bell pepper

Red bell pepper

Yellow bell pepper

Jicama

Red onion

High-hydro fruit option: 1 medium orange

High-hydro protein option: 1 cup rinsed and drained black beans

Herb option: Cilantro

Salsa Dressing (page 192)

BUILD A WRAP

There's nothing like wrapping up an HD-friendly protein or a high-hydro bean spread with high-hydro veggies to go. The best thing about a wrap is you need no utensils! If you don't want to use a carbohydrate, using a nori or collard green wrapper is a great decision. Here are the general HD guidelines for high-hydro veggies.

WRAPPERS

HD-friendly carbohydrate wrap (I like La Tortilla Factory's low-carb ones)

Nori seaweed wrap

Collard green leaf

FILLINGS

HD-friendly protein (4 ounces for women, 6 ounces for men)

High-hydro bean spread (½ cup)

High-hydro vegetables

HIGH-HYDRO VEGETABLE ADD-INS

Whatever else you add, always stuff a wrap with high-hydro vegetables. A chicken wrap with iceberg lettuce, tomatoes, and mustard does not have the same satiating benefits as a wrap filled with high-hydro veggies.

I love using the julienne cutter to prepare many of these veggie stuffers. Thin veggie slices make the wrap easier to roll up. Try all of these high-hydro veggies to find which ones you like best.

Bell peppers, in strips
Broccoli, steamed and chopped
Broccolini, steamed
Cabbage, shredded
Carrots, shredded
Jicama strips
Kale, shredded and boiled for 5 minutes
Spinach, steamed or raw
Yellow squash, steamed but also delicious raw
Zucchini

Don't forget to keep some premade and already cut wraps in clear plastic containers in the fridge. You will be amazed at all the different ways you start to use them.

HD CRUDITÉ

No surprise, I'm sure, but I am a big fan of crudité. With bean spreads (like hummus) and yogurt dips, it's a favorite snack option on the HD plan. Just keep in mind: There's a high-hydro world beyond carrots, though carrots are fine. But if you're in a rut, here are some other crudité veggies to keep in mind.

Asparagus, blanched
Bell peppers (all types)
Broccoli (can be blanched)
Broccolini (can be blanched)
Carrots
Green beans, blanched
Jicama (instead of celery)
Kohlrabi can be eaten raw; it tastes like cabbage and can be cut into matchsticks
Radishes
Sugar snap peas
Yellow squash
Zucchini
HD-friendly options: Cucumber, celery, fennel, cauliflower, tomatoes, and endives

So how do you blanch vegetables?

1. Bring a pot of water to a boil.
2. Prepare a large bowl of ice water.
3. Meanwhile, rinse, trim, or chop the vegetable being used.
4. Put the veggies in the boiling water for the prescribed time (usually 30 seconds to 2 minutes).
5. Drain the vegetables and rinse with cool water.
6. Pat dry.

WAYS TO PREPARE YOUR VEGGIES

It is no surprise that there is an HD way to prepare your veggies. The following methods are listed here for you. Each one limits additional fat and calories, so you can go for seconds—even thirds. Just pick the high-hydro veggies you are in the market for and decide which way you're going to prep.

HD STEAMING

Steamed vegetables are *so* easy. Many clients roll their eyes at me when I tell them they can't go wrong using steam as a cooking method (I assume that's because it sounds so boring and bland). But steamed veggies don't have to be boring. You can dress them up with any of the unlimited condiments (see page 82) and Good Decisions Dressings (pages 189 to 192).

And when ordering at a restaurant, steamed really is your best bet. This way you don't have to wonder what ingredients—like excess oil, salt, or butter (and probably a combination of all three)—were added to your "healthy" side of high-hydro veggies.

- Choose your high-hydro vegetables from the list in Chapter 5
- Throw in a steam basket and you are done.

HD SAUTÉ

I highly recommend that my clients not use oil when sautéing their veggies at home because oil's calories and fat grams can add up fast, especially when you grab a second serving. Many people believe oil is a necessity for sautéing, but it just isn't! Removing it does not alter the taste at all. Here's how.

- Choose any of the high-hydro vegetables from the list in Chapter 5. (Check out possible combos below.)
- Use water or reduced-sodium vegetable broth to replace the oil.
- Add flavor with onions, leeks, scallions, garlic, or ginger, to name a few. Refer to the unlimited condiments list on page 82 and get creative.

The veggie combinations are endless, but here are a few of my favorites.

Asparagus, carrots, onion, red bell pepper

Broccoli, snow peas, yellow squash

Zucchini, yellow squash, red bell pepper, okra

Jicama, carrots, green beans

HD ROASTING

Roasted high-hydro vegetables are so satisfying! That's because roasted veggies become caramelized on the outside, adding so much flavor. It's really a great way to get your high-hydros in. Of course, I caution against dousing the veggies in oil, even olive oil. Here are some HD roasting tips.

- Don't oil the bottom of the roasting pan. Add a little water or reduced-sodium broth instead.
- Place vegetables in the pan and mist with olive oil spray for just 4 to 5 seconds.
- If they do not seem wet enough, put more reduced-sodium broth on top. Other options include lemon juice, rice vinegar, or balsamic vinegar.
- Do not forget to season. Some wonderful options are garlic powder, thyme, dried fennel, or sage.

HD MASHES

I do love my hand blender. It's wonderful for mashing your vegetables, and mashed vegetables are a great way to experience your high-hydro veggies. I use the hand blender for mashing carrots, broccoli, and turnips. Add 1 to 2 tablespoons of Chia Gel (page 158) to give these veggies a hydro-boost plus added thickness.

LIZ, 34, *Lost 25 Pounds*

Before HD: I was at my heaviest—over 250 pounds. I drive a lot for my job, so I was pretty much eating whatever I could take with me in the car. I decided this was crazy and that I really needed to start making changes.

Starting strong: Eating vegetables and more raw nutrients wasn't hard. For me, it was more about learning to eat proper portions and cutting out milk. My dairy intake was pretty high, so switching over to almond milk helped. I liked the HD plan because I just wanted to know which foods were okay to eat and not worry about numbers or points or feel that I was "done" for the day. There has to be something that's okay to eat to get you through those hunger pangs.

New foods: Almond milk. Chia seeds (they're such an easy addition, and I like what they're doing for me). Bean sprouts. Shirataki noodles. Zucchini "Fettuccini."

Unexpected bonus: Foods like the Decision Nutrition Chia Chips. You don't feel very guilty eating them, and they keep you feeling fuller longer! Also, oatmeal with chia and cinnamon and berries—I love berries—instead of a boxed sugar cereal in the morning. It keeps me fuller for longer.

Lesson learned: It's not about avoiding carbs; it's about learning which carbs are better. The HD plan has also made me aware of how much protein I was eating. I thought I was doing good—adding chicken and beans to my salad!—but Keren helped me realize I was overportioning. I fine-tuned my approach and it worked.

Liz really started to focus on high-hydro carbohydrate options. She had been eating a lot of refined carbohydrates during the day, which would start a vicious cycle of eating. She also really took control of her portions once she started eating foods that filled her up, instead of filling her out!

New mantra: Don't satiate your hunger with foods that aren't HD. Every day you have to make the choice.

Sustaining in HD: I'm the mother of two girls and a Girl Scout leader. This keeps me very busy, and every weekend there's a function or a kid's birthday party with pizza and soda and food laid out. So in the beginning, it was very hard for me, but Keren said, "Liz, it's an hour and a half of your day." So now I prepare myself a little bit more.

Inspiring words: I'm so much more aware of when I'm starting to get full than I was in the past.

11

THE **HD RECIPES**

Let me begin by saying I'm not a professional chef. In fact, the simplicity of the HD "Cheat Sheet" (page 90) is really my family's speed. But there is nothing wrong with expanding your culinary repertoire, and I hope these recipes get you thinking about new ways to "live HD" in your kitchen. You know by now that I'm not too keen on salt, but feel free to add salt and pepper to taste.

There are also many recipes that call for a light coat of cooking spray. Please keep the cooking spray guidelines from page 83 in mind when using it. Four seconds is equivalent to around 40 calories. That is all you need!

BREAKFAST

APPLE-CINNAMON OATMEAL

MAKES 2 SERVINGS

I love the taste of apple pie filling. That's what this recipe reminds me of. It is a breakfast that starts the day off right, and it is simply delicious!

1 cup rolled oats

1 cup water

1 cup unsweetened almond milk

1 apple, cut into small cubes (Do not peel! Remember the peel contains a lot of hydrophilic fiber)

⅛ teaspoon ground cinnamon

½ teaspoon vanilla extract

Stevia to taste (optional)

In a medium saucepan over medium-high heat, combine the oats, water, almond milk, apple, cinnamon, and vanilla and bring to a boil, stirring occasionally.

Reduce the heat to low and cook for 10 minutes, or until the oats and apple are soft. Remove from the heat and sweeten with stevia, if using.

QUICK CHIA OATMEAL

MAKES 1 SERVING

We all have those days when we just can't think. So have your instant oatmeal packets ready! As long as there is no added sugar (sorry, no maple and brown sugar oatmeal), you can have a delicious filling breakfast. Both the Quick Chia Oatmeal and Quick Cacao Oatmeal are amazing with your choice of high-hydro berries (fresh or frozen).

- 1 packet plain instant oatmeal or ⅓ cup instant oats
- 1 tablespoon chia seeds
- ¼ cup unsweetened almond milk
- ¼ teaspoon vanilla extract (optional)
- Stevia to taste (optional)

Cook the oatmeal according to package directions. Add the chia seeds, almond milk, and vanilla and stevia (if using) and combine.

QUICK CACAO CHIA OATMEAL:

Add 1 teaspoon raw cacao powder.

WHILE-YOU-SLEEP CHIA OATMEAL

MAKES 1 SERVING

I love this recipe because you can prepare it the night before your anticipated busy morning. All you do is wake up and your oatmeal is the perfect consistency. You can enjoy it cold or, if you prefer, heated up. It's delicious either way. If you feel like having fruit, add any high-hydro option from the list on page 72 (my faves are strawberries and blueberries).

½ cup rolled oats

1 cup unsweetened vanilla almond milk

1 tablespoon chia seeds

¼ teaspoon ground cinnamon

1 teaspoon vanilla extract

In a small plastic container or mason jar, add the oats, almond milk, chia seeds, cinnamon, and vanilla. Cover with a tight-fitting lid and shake until combined.

Refrigerate overnight. In the morning, eat the oatmeal cold or heat it up.

BARLEY BREAKFAST

MAKES 4 SERVINGS (½ CUP EACH)

This breakfast can be made with any high-hydro grain, but barley is my favorite (besides oats). It's a great way to change it up once in a while.

½ cup pearled barley

1 cup unsweetened vanilla almond milk

1½ cups water

½ teaspoon ground cinnamon

Stevia to taste (optional)

In a medium saucepan over high heat, combine the barley, almond milk, water, and cinnamon and bring to a boil.

Reduce the heat to low, cover, and simmer for 30 to 40 minutes, or until all the liquid is absorbed. Remove from the heat and sweeten with stevia, if using.

BRUSSELS EGG SCRAMBLE

MAKES 2 SERVINGS

Scrambled eggs are a breakfast favorite. On the HD plan, it is essential to add a high-hydro vegetable with an HD-friendly protein. I love starting my day with these eggs!

2 eggs and 4 egg whites, or 10 egg whites

¼ red onion, chopped

1 clove garlic, minced

15 Brussels sprouts, stems removed and sliced

In a medium bowl, beat the eggs and set aside.

In a large nonstick skillet lightly coated with cooking spray over medium heat, cook the onion for 10 minutes, or until translucent. Add the garlic and cook for 30 seconds, stirring constantly. Add the Brussels sprouts and cook for 5 minutes, or until soft and caramelized.

Pour in the reserved eggs and scramble for 3 minutes, or until the eggs are set.

CHIA-OAT PANCAKE

MAKES 1 SERVING

Sometimes you just want a pancake. This healthy, HD-satiating version is really yummy.

1/3 cup instant oats

1/3 cup egg whites (2–3 egg whites)

1/2 teaspoon baking powder

1/2 teaspoon vanilla extract

1 tablespoon chia seeds

1/4 teaspoon ground cinnamon

In a medium bowl, mix together the oats, egg whites, baking powder, vanilla, chia seeds, and cinnamon.

Heat a medium nonstick skillet lightly coated with cooking spray over medium heat. Pour in the batter while shaping it into a large disk with a spoon. Cook for 2 minutes, or until you can shake the pancake around in the pan. Flip and cook for 2 minutes, or until cooked through.

Note: Top the pancake with any high-hydro fruit option on page 72 or Chia-Raspberry Smash (page 185).

EGGSELLENT OMELET

MAKES 1 SERVING

1 egg and 2 egg whites, or 5 egg whites

3 tablespoons Chia Gel (page 158; optional)

1 cup high-hydro vegetable of choice (my favorite is steamed broccoli or raw spinach)

In a medium bowl, whisk the eggs with a fork. Mix in the gel, if using.

In a medium nonstick skillet lightly coated with cooking spray over medium heat, cook the egg mixture for 5 minutes, or until set.

Place the high-hydro veggies in the center and fold the omelet in half. Cover and cook for 3 minutes, or until cooked through.

MICROWAVE CHIA EGG SOUFFLÉ

MAKES 1 SERVING

This recipe comes from the only meal my dad ever made my sister and me—Microwave Cheese Egg Soufflé (that's what he called it). It really was delicious, and the eggs would fluff up just like a soufflé. Of course, I wanted to make it HD-plan worthy, so I added high-hydro vegetables and hydro-booster chia seeds and removed the cheese. This is a quick, easy morning option.

- 1 egg and 2 egg whites, or 5 egg whites
- ¼ cup chopped red bell pepper
- ½ cup chopped zucchini
- 1 tablespoon chia seeds
- 1 tablespoon water

In a medium bowl, combine the eggs, bell pepper, zucchini, chia seeds, and water and beat thoroughly.

Pour into an 8-ounce ramekin lightly coated with cooking spray. Cover (I just use a microwaveable plate) and microwave on high power for 2 minutes and 30 seconds, or until cooked through.

Pop out and serve!

SWISS CHARD MINI FRITTATAS

MAKES 3 SERVINGS (2 MINI FRITTATAS PER SERVING)

This mini frittata works well with spinach and kale, too. The great thing is you can save the extra servings for a quick grab-and-go breakfast during the week or as an HD-friendly protein/high-hydro vegetable snack.

½ onion, chopped

1 clove garlic, minced

3 eggs and 6 egg whites

½ bunch Swiss chard, stems removed and finely chopped

½ teaspoon kelp powder

½ teaspoon ground black pepper

Preheat the oven to 350°F. Lightly coat a 6-cup muffin pan with cooking spray.

In a medium saucepan over medium heat, add a splash of water (just enough to wet the saucepan) and cook the onion and garlic, stirring frequently, for a few minutes, or until the onion is translucent.

In a large bowl, beat the eggs thoroughly, so that the yolks are completely broken up and incorporated in the whites. Add the onion mixture, Swiss chard, kelp powder, and pepper and mix well.

Divide the egg mixture evenly among the muffin cups (cups will be two-thirds full). Bake for 25 minutes, or until brown on top. Let cool for 10 minutes.

TOFU SCRAMBLER

MAKES 4 SERVINGS

This is a delicious snack or meal to put on crackers or eat alone.

2 tablespoons nutritional yeast

1 tablespoon onion powder

½ teaspoon curry powder

½ teaspoon ground turmeric

½ teaspoon ground cumin

3 tablespoons water

1 package reduced-fat, extra-firm tofu, drained and pressed

1 cup spinach

In a small bowl, combine the nutritional yeast, onion powder, curry powder, turmeric, cumin, and water and set aside.

In a medium nonstick skillet lightly coated with cooking spray over medium heat, break apart the tofu and cook for 10 minutes, or until heated through.

Add the reserved spice mixture and combine thoroughly. Add the spinach and stir until wilted.

DIPS AND SPREADS

YOGURT DIP

MAKES 1 SERVING

Who doesn't like some creamy dip with their veggies? I love making an individual container of plain Greek yogurt into my own personal dip to plunge my high-hydro veggies in. The portion is an entire container, so you can really enjoy.

These dips taste best when refrigerated for at least 1 hour. It may take some preplanning, but it's worth it. Oh, and remember to look over the HD Crudité options on page 165.

ALWAYS START WITH:

1 container (6 ounces) 0% plain Greek yogurt

ONION YOGURT DIP

¼ teaspoon garlic powder

1 teaspoon onion powder

1 teaspoon kelp powder

1 tablespoon Chia Gel (page 158; optional)

HORSERADISH YOGURT DIP

1 tablespoon prepared horseradish

2 tablespoons lemon juice

½ teaspoon grated lemon peel

1 tablespoon Chia Gel (page 158; optional)

DILL YOGURT DIP

1 tablespoon chopped fresh dill

1 clove garlic, minced

1 tablespoon lemon juice

1 tablespoon Chia Gel (page 158; optional)

Once you decide what you are in the mood for, put all the ingredients in a small mixing bowl and combine thoroughly. Cover and refrigerate for at least 1 hour.

CHICKPEA SPREAD

MAKES 4 SERVINGS (½ CUP EACH)

This high-hydro protein spread is amazing on sandwiches or as a vegetable dip. The same is true for all the bean dips.

1 can (14–19 ounces) no-salt-added chickpeas with liquid (see note)

¼ cup shredded carrot

1 clove garlic, minced

3 tablespoons Chia Gel (page 158)

2 tablespoons Good Decisions Dressing (pages 189 to 192; I love the miso one) or any vinegar (rice wine vinegar is good)

1 tablespoon lemon juice

In a large mixing bowl, combine the chickpeas, carrot, garlic, gel, and dressing and mix with a hand blender until smooth.

Cover and refrigerate for up to 2 days.

Note: Instead of canned, you can cook your own beans from scratch. See page 159 for tips on how to cook dried beans.

CHIA NUT BUTTER

MAKES 1 SERVING (1/4 CUP)

This is a way to get your hydroboost in either your peanut or almond butter and get more delicious nut butter in one serving for less calories and fat. It's easy!

1 tablespoon natural almond or peanut butter

3 tablespoons of chia gel (page 158)

In a medium mixing bowl, combine the nut butter and chia gel, mix thoroughly, and serve. You can make this to save and use later as well.

WHITE BEAN DIP

MAKES 4 SERVINGS (½ CUP EACH)

- 1 can (14–19 ounces) no-salt-added cannellini beans, rinsed and drained (see note on page 183)
- 1½ teaspoons garlic powder
- 1½ tablespoons lemon juice
- ½ teaspoon paprika
- 1 tablespoon chia seeds
- 2 tablespoons water

In a large mixing bowl, combine the beans, garlic powder, lemon juice, paprika, and chia seeds. With a hand blender, puree while adding the water until smooth.

Cover and refrigerate for up to 2 days.

BLACK BEAN DIP

MAKES 4 SERVINGS (½ CUP EACH)

- 1 can (14–19 ounces) no-salt-added black beans, rinsed and drained (see note on page 183)
- ½ cup salsa
- 2 tablespoons lemon juice
- 2 tablespoons chopped fresh cilantro
- ¼ teaspoon ground cumin
- 1 tablespoon chia seeds (optional)

In a large mixing bowl, combine the beans, salsa, lemon juice, cilantro, cumin, and chia seeds (if using) and mix with a hand blender until smooth.

Cover and refrigerate for up to 2 days.

EDAMAME DIP

MAKES 4 SERVINGS (½ CUP EACH)

1 pound frozen shelled edamame, thawed

2 cloves garlic, minced

1 tablespoon lemon juice

3 tablespoons Chia Gel (page 158)

¼ cup rice wine vinegar

In a large mixing bowl, combine the edamame, garlic, lemon juice, gel, and vinegar and mix with a hand blender until smooth.

Cover and refrigerate for up to 2 days.

CHIA-RASPBERRY SMASH

MAKES 2 SERVINGS

This jam is delicious with strawberries and blueberries, too! Use as a topping for the Chia-Oat Pancake on page 177, with nut butters, or swirled into yogurt or oatmeal.

1 cup frozen raspberries, thawed

2 tablespoons chia seeds

2 stevia packets

2 tablespoons water

Place the raspberries in a medium microwaveable bowl. Microwave on high power for 45 seconds, or until easy to mash.

Mash the mixture with a fork. Add the chia seeds, stevia, and water and stir to combine.

Pour the raspberry mixture into a mason jar, cover tightly with the lid, and refrigerate for at least 1 hour.

SALADS AND DRESSINGS

Since the next three salads are made with high-hydro vegetables and "unlimited" condiments (see page 82), feel free to go for seconds.

ARAME AND KALE SALAD

MAKES 2 SERVINGS

1 big bunch kale, stems removed and chopped
2 teaspoons Bragg Liquid Aminos
1 teaspoon lemon juice
cup dried arame, soaked in cold water for 15 minutes and drained
1–2 teaspoons sesame seeds

In a large nonstick skillet over medium heat, warm a small amount of water (just enough to cover the bottom) and add the kale. Cover and let steam for 2 to 3 minutes, or until bright green. Drain in a colander and set aside.

In a medium bowl, combine the Bragg Liquid Aminos and lemon juice. Add the steamed kale and toss. Add the arame and mix well. Sprinkle with the sesame seeds.

Serve while still warm, or chill the salad in the refrigerator and eat cold.

ASPARAGUS AND ARTICHOKE SALAD

MAKES 2 SERVINGS

1 bag (9 ounces) frozen artichoke hearts

1 pound asparagus, ends cut off and discarded

½ red onion, sliced

2 cups cherry tomatoes, halved

3 tablespoons lemon juice

Cook the artichoke hearts according to package directions and set aside.

Place a steamer basket in a large pot of water. Bring to a boil over high heat. Steam the asparagus in the basket for 5 minutes, or until fork-tender.

In a large bowl, combine the reserved artichokes, asparagus, onion, tomatoes, and lemon juice.

BROCCOLI–RED CABBAGE SLAW

MAKES 2 LARGE SERVINGS

This recipe is wonderful with chopped apples if you want to use a high-hydro fruit. It's also great topped with sesame seeds or pumpkin seeds.

1 package broccoli slaw

½ head cabbage, thinly sliced

⅓ cup red wine vinegar

2 tablespoons lemon juice

2 tablespoons Chia Gel (page 158)

2 packets stevia

In a large bowl, combine the broccoli slaw and cabbage.

In a separate bowl, add the vinegar, lemon juice, gel, and stevia and whisk with a fork. Pour into the slaw mix and combine.

Cover and refrigerate for 1 hour.

GOOD DECISIONS DRESSINGS

MAKES 2 SERVINGS

All the HD dressings contain Chia Gel to replace oil. A good dressing requires a good sliminess, which oil usually provides, but Chia Gel does the trick. You can eliminate the gel if you desire, though, and the dressings will still taste good. And since there is no oil in any of these dressings, feel free to use as much as you desire. All dressings can be stored in a mason jar for up to a week.

BALSAMIC MUSTARD DRESSING

This is my basic go-to dressing. It's good to have on hand for the Ultimate HD Salads you make at home.

¼ cup balsamic vinegar

¼ cup water

1 tablespoon Dijon mustard

2 cloves garlic, minced

3 tablespoons Chia Gel (page 158; optional)

In a large bowl, combine the vinegar, water, mustard, and garlic. Slowly pour in the gel, if using, and mix with a hand blender until the desired consistency.

LEMON-OREGANO DRESSING

This is so refreshing and clean tasting. I can eat salad with just a squeeze of lemon juice and be satisfied, but this dressing has more oomph.

¼ cup fresh lemon juice

2 tablespoons apple cider vinegar

2 teaspoons Dijon mustard

1 clove garlic, minced

2 teaspoons dried oregano

1 packet stevia

3 tablespoons Chia Gel (page 158; optional)

In a large bowl, whisk together the lemon juice, vinegar, mustard, garlic, oregano, and stevia. Slowly pour in the gel, if using, and mix with a hand blender until the desired consistency.

MISO DRESSING

I love this dressing on the Ultimate HD Salad with Asian Flair (page 164), but you can use it on any salad you build in HD. I also love using it in the Chickpea Spread (page 183) because it adds thickness and flavor. You can give it a try as a sauce on chicken or fish, too. I highly recommend using the Chia Gel in this recipe. It makes it so thick and creamy (as does using the hand blender). You won't believe there is no oil in it!

¼ cup unsweetened almond milk

1 teaspoon miso paste (white or dark)

1 tablespoon rice wine vinegar

2 scallions, chopped

1 tablespoon reduced-sodium tamari or Bragg Liquid Aminos

3 tablespoons Chia Gel (page 158; optional)

In a large bowl, combine the almond milk, miso paste, vinegar, scallions, and tamari. Slowly pour in the gel, if using, and mix with a hand blender until the desired consistency.

SALSA DRESSING

I always use store-brought salsa for this recipe because it's fast and easy. I like Green Mountain Gringo (it's low in sodium). This dressing is delicious on the Ultimate HD Salad with Latin Flair (page 164), but you can also use it to flavor your high-hydro vegetables or wraps.

½ cup salsa

2 tablespoons lemon juice

1 tablespoon rice wine vinegar

1 tablespoon chopped fresh cilantro

1 clove garlic, minced

3 tablespoons Chia Gel (page 158; optional)

In a large bowl, combine the salsa, lemon juice, vinegar, cilantro, and garlic. Slowly pour in the gel, if using, and mix with a hand blender until the desired consistency.

SOUPS AND SIDES

BROCCOLI SOUP*

MAKES 6 SERVINGS

This soup is especially terrific during the Start Strong phase. I tell my clients that because it's an HD freebie. Keep this soup on hand so you can just heat some up whenever hunger pangs hit and get HD-satiated right away.

2 cups reduced-sodium chicken broth or vegetable broth

2 cups water

2 heads broccoli, chopped

3 carrots, sliced

1 small onion, cut into rings

1 teaspoon kelp powder

In a large pot over high heat, combine the broth, water, broccoli, carrots, onion, and kelp powder and bring to a boil. Reduce the heat to low and simmer for 30 minutes, or until the vegetables are tender.

Puree the soup with a hand blender for a creamier outcome!

*This is on the freebie list in Chapter 6 (page 106) so if you want seconds—go for it!

GAZPACHO SOUP*

MAKES 6 SERVINGS

You can use 2 cans (14.5 ounces each) of diced tomatoes instead of fresh in this recipe if you want to save time. Just make sure they have no added salt. Add a serving of steamed shrimp or crabmeat as an HD-friendly protein. This is an HD freebie, so have a bowl whenever the urge strikes!

- 4–6 tomatoes
- 1 small red onion, chopped
- 1 zucchini, chopped
- 1 red bell pepper, chopped
- 1 clove garlic, minced
- 2 tablespoons chopped fresh parsley
- 2 tablespoons chopped fresh basil
- 2 tablespoons chopped fresh cilantro
- 5 cups reduced-sodium tomato juice
- 2 tablespoons lemon juice
- 2 tablespoons balsamic vinegar
- 1 teaspoon finely chopped chives

Bring a large pot of water to a boil. Cook the tomatoes for 30 seconds. Drain and let cool. Peel the skin away and dice. Return the tomatoes to the empty pot.

Add the onion, zucchini, bell pepper, garlic, parsley, basil, cilantro, tomato juice, lemon juice, vinegar, and chives and stir until evenly combined. Mix with a hand blender until the desired consistency.

Cover and refrigerate for at least 3 hours.

*This is on the freebie list in Chapter 6 (page 106) so if you want seconds—go for it!

GOOD DECISIONS SOUP*

MAKES 10 SERVINGS

I love this soup and encourage my clients to make it at the beginning of the week to have for the whole week. It can be stored in the fridge for up to 5 days, and 2-cup portions can be kept in the freezer for up to 1 month. Like the Broccoli Soup (page 193) and Gazpacho Soup (page 194), this is an HD freebie, so heat some up whenever you need to feel HD satiated. I put a lot of high-hydro veggies in this soup, but you can decide which ones you want to use if not all of them.

1 onion, chopped

4 cloves garlic, minced

3 ribs celery, chopped

1 package (8 ounces) mushrooms

8 cups reduced-sodium vegetable broth or chicken broth

1 pound okra, chopped

1 cup sliced carrots

1 zucchini, chopped

2 cups chopped broccoli

1 cup chopped cauliflower

3 cups roughly chopped cabbage

1 can (14.5 ounces) no-salt-added diced tomatoes

2 bay leaves

2 tablespoons apple cider vinegar

In a large pot lightly coated with cooking spray over medium heat, cook the onion, garlic, celery, and mushrooms, stirring occasionally, for 10 minutes, or until tender.

Add the broth, okra, carrots, zucchini, broccoli, cauliflower, cabbage, tomatoes, and bay leaves and bring to a boil. Reduce the heat to low, cover, and simmer for 20 minutes, or until the vegetables are tender throughout.

Add the vinegar and cook for 1 minute. Discard the bay leaves and serve. Allow the soup to cool to room temperature before storing.

*This is on the freebie list in Chapter 6 (page 106) so if you want seconds—go for it!

LENTIL SOUP

MAKES 4 SERVINGS

Unlike the Broccoli Soup (page 193) and the Good Decisions Soup (page 195), bean soups are never unlimited. Watch your portion sizes! If you're enjoying it as a starter, have 1 serving and count it as a high-hydro carb. If you're having it as a main meal, have 2 servings and count it as a high-hydro protein.

1 cup dried lentils, soaked in warm water for 20 minutes, rinsed, and drained

2 onions, chopped

3 cups reduced-sodium vegetable broth

4 carrots, chopped

1 rib celery, chopped

1 teaspoon reduced-sodium tamari or Bragg Liquid Aminos

1 cup chopped fresh spinach

In a large pot over medium heat, combine the lentils, onions, and broth and bring to a boil. Reduce the heat to low, cover, and simmer for 15 minutes, or until the lentils are tender.

Add the carrots and celery and cook for 30 minutes, or until tender.

Stir in the tamari or Bragg Liquid Aminos and spinach.

Note: If you want to add a high-hydro carbohydrate, 1 cup cubed butternut squash is delicious in this soup.

LIMA BEAN–OKRA SOUP

MAKES 6 SERVINGS

Again, if you're having this as a starter, keep the portion to ½ serving and count it as a high-hydro carb. If it's your main meal, 1 serving counts as a high-hydro protein.

- 1 green bell pepper, chopped
- 1 scallion, chopped
- 2 cloves garlic, minced
- 1 bag (16 ounces) frozen and thawed lima beans
- 3 cups fresh or frozen and thawed sliced okra
- 3 cups reduced-sodium vegetable broth
- 4 tomatoes, chopped
- ½ cup fresh or frozen and thawed peas

Lightly coat a large pot with cooking spray and place over medium heat. Add the bell pepper, scallion, and garlic and cook until the peppers soften.

Stir in the lima beans, okra, broth, tomatoes, and peas and bring to a boil. Reduce the heat to low and simmer for 20 minutes, or until the lima beans are tender.

VEGETABLE-CHIA MISO SOUP*

MAKES 4 SERVINGS

You can have this soup whenever you want. It's on the freebie list on page 106. It's very comforting, filling, and good for you. Shortcut! If you are feeling lazy, buy a reduced-sodium prepared miso pack, follow the package directions, and add 2 tablespoons Chia Gel and steamed high-hydro veggies to your bowl.

3 cups water

1 tablespoon miso paste (white or dark)

2 scallions, chopped

1 bunch broccoli, chopped

2 carrots, chopped

2 tablespoons Chia Gel (page 158)

¼ cup seaweed (like wakame or kelp), soaked in cold water for 15 minutes and drained

In a large pot over high heat, add the water, miso paste, scallions, broccoli, and carrots and mix well. Bring to a boil.

Reduce the heat to medium-low and add the gel and seaweed. Cover and simmer for 20 minutes, or until the vegetables are the desired consistency.

*This is on the freebie list in Chapter 6 (page 106) so if you want seconds—go for it!

TURKEY CHILI

MAKES 4 SERVINGS

There is nothing more comforting and filling than a big bowl of chili. The beans in this dish count as a high-hydro carbohydrate since an HD-friendly protein is used, but it's worth it. If you want to save your carbs, take the turkey out and add another can of beans. Serve 1½ cups with an Ultimate HD Salad (page 161) for dinner.

- 1 red onion, chopped
- 1 clove garlic, minced
- 1 pound lean ground turkey
- ½ cup reduced-sodium vegetable broth
- 2 cans (14.5 ounces each) no-salt-added diced tomatoes
- 1 can (14–19 ounces) no-salt-added kidney beans, rinsed and drained (see note on page 183)
- 1 can (8 ounces) reduced-sugar tomato sauce
- 1 tablespoon ground cumin
- 2 teaspoons chili powder (optional)
- ⅛ teaspoon ground cinnamon

In a large pot coated with cooking spray over medium heat, cook the onion and garlic, stirring frequently, for 5 minutes, or until translucent.

Add the ground turkey and cook for 15 minutes, or until no longer pink.

Add the broth, tomatoes, beans, tomato sauce, cumin, chili powder (if using), and cinnamon and mix well. Bring to a boil.

Reduce the heat to low and simmer for 20 minutes, or until the turkey is cooked through.

HD RATATOUILLE

MAKES 6 SERVINGS

This is a comfort meal that is filled with high-hydro vegetables. I love it with eggplant, which doesn't have so much hydrophilic fiber, but I make up for it by adding okra. This ratatouille is amazing on its own, but it can also be combined with a high-hydro protein (like chickpeas) or an HD-friendly protein (like grilled chicken or fish) and a high-hydro carbohydrate, like brown rice. I love saving the leftovers and using them in a wrap the next day.

¼ cup reduced-sodium vegetable broth

3 tablespoons Chia Gel (page 158; optional)

3 cloves garlic, minced

1 onion, sliced

1 pound okra, sliced

2 zucchini, cut into ½-inch-thick slices

1 large red bell pepper, chopped

2 large eggplant, cut into ½-inch cubes

2 cans (14.5 ounces each) no-salt-added diced tomatoes

1 tablespoon fresh basil

1 tablespoon finely chopped fresh thyme or 2 teaspoons dried

In a large pot over medium heat, cook the broth, gel (if using), garlic, onion, okra, zucchini, and pepper, stirring occasionally, for 10 minutes or until you can pierce easily with a knife.

Add the eggplant, tomatoes, basil, and thyme. Reduce the heat to low, cover, and cook for 40 minutes, or until the eggplant is tender.

MASHED TURNIPS

MAKES 2 SERVINGS

This is a great replacement for mashed potatoes. And turnips are a high-hydro vegetable, which makes this a wonderful side dish. It's delicious with a side of sliced turkey breast and high-hydro veggies roasted the HD way (page 167). This dish is so easy to make, and you will feel like it's Thanksgiving on a random weeknight.

- 3 cups peeled and cubed turnips (about 2 large)
- ½ cup unsweetened almond milk
- 1 teaspoon garlic powder
- Salt to taste

Bring a large pot of water to a boil. Cook the turnips for 20 minutes, or until tender.

Drain and put back in the pot. Pour in the almond milk and garlic powder while mixing with a hand blender until smooth. Add salt to taste.

PARSNIP FRIES

MAKES 2 SERVINGS

2 tablespoons reduced-sodium vegetable broth

1 teaspoon garlic powder

2 teaspoons dried oregano

2 parsnips, peeled and cut lengthwise into long strips

Preheat the oven to 450°F. Line a baking sheet with parchment paper.

In a medium bowl, combine the broth, garlic powder, and oregano. Add the parsnips and coat well.

Place the parsnips on the baking sheet and lightly coat with cooking spray. Bake for 15 minutes, or until the fries begin to brown at the edges. Turn over and cook for 15 minutes, or until tender.

SPAGHETTI SQUASH

MAKES 2 SERVINGS

As mentioned in Chapter 6, spaghetti squash is a carb fake-out, so I like to think of it as the real Italian pasta we all crave. I encourage you to add other cooked high-hydro veggies (like zucchini, broccoli, or asparagus) to this recipe for a "pasta" primavera dish.

1 spaghetti squash, halved lengthwise and seeds removed

1 cup marinara sauce

Preheat the oven to 450°F. Line a baking sheet with foil.

Lightly coat the squash with cooking spray. Place flesh side down on the baking sheet and roast for 30 to 40 minutes, or until fully cooked. Remove and allow to cool.

Meanwhile, in a large saucepan over medium heat, warm the marinara sauce.

When the squash is cool enough to handle, scrape the strands from the inside of the skin with a large kitchen spoon. Toss the squash in the saucepan with the warmed marinara for just long enough to get hot.

SWEET POTATO FRIES

MAKES 4 SERVINGS

Here is a way to have fries with no oil. They are delicious!

- 2 sweet potatoes, cut lengthwise into long, narrow strips (Do not peel!)
- Spices of choice to taste (paprika, garlic powder, ground red pepper, or ground cinnamon are all good decisions)

Preheat the oven to 350°F. Line a baking sheet with parchment paper.

Place the sweet potatoes on the baking sheet and add the spices to taste. Bake for 30 minutes, flipping once halfway through baking.

Change the setting to broil and broil for 15 minutes, or until the tops are browned.

SWEET POTATO ROAST

MAKES 4 SERVINGS

- 2 sweet potatoes, cut into wedges (Do not peel!)
- 1 onion, chopped
- ¼ cup reduced-sodium vegetable broth
- Seasonings of choice to taste (great with paprika, dried rosemary, or dried thyme)
- 3 tablespoons Chia Gel (page 158; optional)

Preheat the oven to 375°F.

In a large baking pan, combine the sweet potatoes, onion, broth, seasonings, and gel, if using. Cook for 45 to 50 minutes, or until tender.

ZUCCHINI "FETTUCCINE"

MAKES 2 SERVINGS

This dish is a great pasta substitute. Just watch your sauce portioning—too much and you'll undo some of the high-hydro benefits.

3 zucchini, cut into strips using the julienne cutter

1 tablespoon sea salt

1 onion, finely chopped

4 cloves garlic, minced

1 cup pasta sauce (I love Rao's)

3 large tomatoes, chopped

Place the zucchini in a colander and sprinkle with the salt. After 20 minutes, rinse thoroughly and pat dry with paper towels.

In a large nonstick skillet lightly coated with cooking spray over medium heat, cook the onion and garlic, stirring occasionally, for a few minutes, or until the onion is translucent.

Add the pasta sauce and tomatoes and cook for 10 minutes. Add the zucchini and cook for 5 minutes, or until the desired tenderness.

ENTRÉES

BEAN-STUFFED ACORN SQUASH

MAKES 2 SERVINGS

1 acorn squash, halved

1 onion, chopped

¼ cup reduced-sodium vegetable broth

1 can (14–19 ounces) white beans, rinsed and drained (see note on page 183)

1 cup chopped fresh spinach

1 teaspoon chopped fresh sage

1 teaspoon chopped fresh thyme

6 tablespoons Chia Gel (page 158)

Preheat the oven to 400°F.

Lightly coat the squash with cooking spray. Place cut sides down on a baking pan lined with foil and roast for 30 minutes, or until tender. Flip over and set aside.

Meanwhile, in a medium saucepan over medium heat, cook the onion with the broth, stirring occasionally, for 5 minutes, or until the onion is translucent.

Add the beans, spinach, sage, thyme, and gel and cook for 3 minutes, or until the spinach wilts.

Divide the bean stuffing evenly among the reserved squash halves and roast for 20 minutes.

BALSAMIC CHICKEN

MAKES 4 SERVINGS

Remember that the serving size for an HD-friendly protein is 4 ounces for women and 6 ounces for men, so buy your cuts of chicken according to which size(s) you need.

¼ cup reduced-sodium vegetable broth

4 boneless, skinless chicken breast halves

2 cups cherry tomatoes, halved

2 yellow squash, chopped

2 cloves garlic, minced

½ cup balsamic vinegar

4 tablespoons chopped fresh basil

3 tablespoons Chia Gel (page 158)

In a large nonstick skillet over medium heat, warm the broth. Add the chicken and cook for a few minutes, turning once, or until cooked through. Transfer to a large plate and set aside.

In the same skillet, cook the tomatoes, squash, and garlic for 1 to 2 minutes. Add the vinegar, basil, and gel and cook for 1 minute.

Pour the squash mixture over the reserved chicken breasts.

CINNAMON CHICKEN

MAKES 2 SERVINGS

This chicken dish is great served over an HD salad or with your choice of a high-hydro carbohydrate. A baked sweet potato is a great option (remember that a sweet potato should be cut to fill just one-quarter of your plate!)

½ teaspoon ground cinnamon

1 clove garlic, minced

2 tablespoons chopped fresh cilantro

2 tablespoons lemon juice

2 tablespoons chia seeds

2 tablespoons water

2 boneless, skinless chicken breast halves, cut into cubes

Preheat the oven to 375°F. Line a baking sheet with parchment paper.

In a large bowl, combine the cinnamon, garlic, cilantro, lemon juice, chia seeds, and water. Add the chicken and mix to coat. Cover and chill for 30 minutes.

Place the chicken pieces 1 inch apart on the baking sheet, shaking off any excess marinade. Bake for 15 minutes, or until cooked through.

LEMON GRILLED CHICKEN

MAKES 2 SERVINGS

This is fast and simple. There is no oil, and you won't even miss it!

1 tablespoon grated lemon peel

2 tablespoons lemon juice

2 teaspoons finely chopped fresh rosemary

2 boneless, skinless chicken breast halves

Preheat the grill to high.

In a small bowl, whisk together the lemon peel, lemon juice, and rosemary.

Place the chicken breast in a shallow bowl. Pour half of the lemon mixture on top of the chicken and marinate for 15 minutes. Set the other half of the lemon mixture aside.

Grill the chicken for 10 minutes on each side, using the reserved lemon mixture to baste the chicken as it grills, until cooked through.

Transfer the chicken breasts to a serving plate.

CABBAGE SPAGHETTI WITH GROUND CHICKEN

MAKES 4 SERVINGS

This dish uses cabbage, but you can use any carb fake-out you like. Cabbage really does the trick, though!

½ onion, chopped

2 cloves garlic, minced

1 pound lean ground chicken

6 cups shredded cabbage

1 red bell pepper, sliced

1 head broccoli, chopped

1 jar (24–32 ounces) reduced-sugar pasta sauce (like Rao's)

In a large nonstick skillet lightly coated with cooking spray over medium heat, cook the onion and garlic for 10 minutes, or until the onion is translucent. Add the ground chicken and cook for 15 minutes, or until no longer pink.

Add the cabbage, pepper, broccoli, and pasta sauce. Cover and cook for 30 minutes, or until the broccoli is tender.

EASY FISH

MAKES 4 SERVINGS

When buying fish, keep the HD portions rule in mind: 4 ounces for women and 6 ounces for men. This dish got its name because it is so easy to prepare. Serve with a high-hydro carbohydrate.

4 whitefish fillets (orange roughy, cod, or halibut)

1 zucchini, cut into strips

1 red bell pepper, sliced

1 fennel bulb, sliced

2 cups cherry tomatoes, halved

2 tablespoons chopped fresh basil

½ cup miso broth or reduced-sodium vegetable broth

Preheat the oven to 350°F. Lay out 4 pieces of foil (each about the length of a forearm).

Place a fillet in the center of each piece of foil. Top evenly with the zucchini, pepper, fennel, tomatoes, and basil. Wet each fillet with the broth.

Fold the foil over the fish tightly. Bake for 20 minutes.

CHIA-CRUSTED SALMON

MAKES 4 SERVINGS

You can use this chia spice mix on chicken or tofu, too. My favorite is salmon, but it's nice to have choices.

- ¼ cup reduced-sodium vegetable broth
- 1 onion, chopped
- ½ cup finely chopped dill
- 4 tablespoons chia seeds
- 4 tablespoons yellow mustard seeds
- 4 salmon fillets

Preheat the broiler.

In a small bowl, combine the broth, onion, and dill and set aside.

In another small bowl, combine the chia seeds and mustard seeds and set aside.

Place the salmon on a baking sheet, skin side down, and broil for 5 minutes, 6 inches from the heat source.

Remove the salmon and pour the broth mixture evenly over the fillets. Broil for 5 minutes.

Remove and coat the fillets with the seed mixture, pressing the seeds into each fillet. Return to the top shelf and broil for 5 to 10 minutes, or until the fish is opaque.

ROSEMARY-LEMON SALMON

MAKES 2 SERVINGS

2 salmon fillets

1 lemon, halved

3 teaspoons finely chopped fresh rosemary

Preheat the oven to 375°F.

Place the fillets, skin side down, in a medium baking dish lightly coated with cooking spray.

Squeeze the lemon juice on the fillets and sprinkle with the rosemary.

Cook for 30 minutes, or until the fish is opaque.

SALMON SALAD NORI WRAP

MAKES 2 SERVINGS

You can also put this salmon salad on top of an Ultimate HD Salad (page 161) as your HD-friendly protein or on an HD-friendly carbohydrate, like quinoa. You can wrap it in a collard green leaf, too, but I love it wrapped in nori the best. You don't use up a carbohydrate, and you get the nutritional benefits of seaweed.

½ jicama, peeled and chopped

½ red onion, chopped

1 tablespoon capers

2 tablespoons lemon juice

1 tablespoon Chia Gel (page 158)

1 can wild salmon, drained (see note)

2 nori wraps

In a large bowl, combine the jicama, onion, capers, lemon juice, and gel. Add the salmon and mix well.

Spread the salmon mixture evenly on the nori wraps and roll up. Best if the wrap is refrigerated for 1 hour.

Note: You can always use a leftover cooked salmon fillet in this recipe instead of canned. Just break apart the salmon until it flakes and mix with the other ingredients.

HD TUNA SALAD

MAKES 2 SERVINGS

- 1 can water-packed tuna, drained
- 2 carrots, finely chopped
- 1 bunch broccolini, steamed and chopped
- ¼ cup peeled and chopped jicama
- 2 tablespoons balsamic vinegar
- 2 tablespoons lemon juice

In a large bowl, combine the tuna, carrots, broccolini, jicama, vinegar, and lemon juice and mix thoroughly.

BAKED TOFU

MAKES 4 SERVINGS

- 1 tablespoon rice wine vinegar or balsamic vinegar
- 1 tablespoon water
- 1 tablespoon reduced-sodium tamari or Bragg Liquid Aminos
- 1–2 packets stevia
- 1 tablespoon minced fresh ginger or ½ teaspoon ground ginger
- 1 tablespoon minced garlic or ½ teaspoon garlic powder
- ½ cup chopped scallions
- ½ teaspoon ground cumin
- ½ teaspoon ground coriander
- Pinch of ground red pepper
- ½ teaspoon ground black pepper
- 1 package (16 ounces) extra-firm tofu, drained, pressed, and cut into ½-inch-thick slices

Place the vinegar, water, tamari, stevia, ginger, garlic, scallions, cumin, coriander, red pepper, and black pepper in a mason jar. Screw the lid on tight and shake until mixed well. Set aside.

Lay the tofu side by side on a baking sheet. Spread the reserved marinade over and under the tofu slices. Cover and marinate for 1 hour in the fridge, turning once or twice, if possible.

Preheat the oven to 375°F.

Drain off the excess marinade. Bake for 40 minutes, flipping the tofu halfway through cooking. (Use a spatula to minimize the chances of the tofu breaking.)

Change the oven temperature to high broil and broil for 5 minutes, or until the tofu has a golden brown crust.

SCALLOP STIR-FRY SHIRATAKI

MAKES 4 SERVINGS

Shirataki noodles taste amazing in stir-fries. You can trick even the pickiest of eaters with this fake-out carb. This dish also works great with tofu, shrimp, or chicken.

- 1 bag angel hair shirataki noodles
- ¼ cup reduced-sodium tamari
- ¼ cup rice wine vinegar
- 3 tablespoons Chia Gel (page 158)
- ¼ cup water
- 2 carrots, chopped
- 1 red bell pepper, sliced
- ½ pound sugar snap peas
- ½ pound green beans, trimmed and chopped
- 1 tablespoon minced garlic
- 1 teaspoon minced fresh ginger
- 1 pound fresh bay scallops
- 1 bunch scallions, chopped

Cook the shirataki noodles according to package directions and set aside.

In a small bowl, whisk together the tamari, vinegar, and gel and set aside.

In a large nonstick skillet over medium-high heat, warm the water. Cook the carrots, pepper, sugar snap peas, green beans, garlic, and ginger, stirring occasionally, for 4 to 5 minutes, or until the carrots begin to soften.

Add the scallops and scallions and cook for 4 to 5 minutes, or until the scallops are opaque.

Add the reserved shirataki and the reserved tamari mixture and combine well.

SPINACH TURKEY BURGERS

MAKES 4 SERVINGS

These burgers are great on top of broccoli slaw.

1 pound lean ground turkey

¾ cup spinach, stems removed and chopped

3 scallions, finely chopped

1 teaspoon onion powder

1 tablespoon tomato paste

1 teaspoon garlic powder

2 tablespoons unsweetened almond milk

Preheat the oven to 375°F.

In a large bowl, combine the ground turkey, spinach, scallions, tomato paste, garlic powder, almond milk, and onion powder and mix thoroughly with a fork.

Make 4 patties and place on a baking sheet lightly coated with cooking spray. Bake for 40 minutes, or until cooked through.

SNACKS

YOGURTS—THE HD WAY

MAKES 1 SERVING

ALWAYS START WITH:

1 container (6 ounces) 0% plain Greek yogurt

BERRY PARFAIT

1 cup high-hydro berries (page 73)

1 tablespoon chia seeds

¼ teaspoon ground cinnamon

Stevia to taste (optional)

BERRY SWIRL YOGURT

4 tablespoons Chia-Raspberry Smash (page 185)

CHIA CACAO YOGURT

This one tastes amazing mixed with a hand blender. It's important to make sure the raw cacao powder is thoroughly distributed.

1 teaspoon raw cacao powder

2 packets stevia

1 tablespoon chia seeds

1 cup raspberries (optional)

Once you decide what you are in the mood for, mix all the ingredients in a medium bowl.

Note: If you are in a rush, you can mix all of the ingredients right into the yogurt container.

AGAR PUDDING*

As you know, agar is on my top 10 list. And after you try these delicious pudding recipes, it will become a favorite ingredient of yours as well! Here you will find the basic recipe for Agar Pudding and then suggested ways to change it up. The chocolate mousse, vanilla, and lemon custard variations are all HD freebies, so enjoy!

2 cups unsweetened vanilla almond milk

2 tablespoons agar flakes

1 tablespoon stevia (see note below)

In a large pot, combine the almond milk, agar flakes, and stevia. Let sit for 5 minutes (the water absorbing process is taking place).

Bring to a boil over high heat. Reduce the heat to medium and simmer, stirring occasionally, for 5 minutes, or until most of the flakes are gone.

Allow to cool for 10 minutes. Cover and refrigerator for at least 1 hour.

Now the fun begins!

Note: If weight loss is not your goal, you can use maple syrup or honey to sweeten.

CHOCOLATE MOUSSE AGAR PUDDING (enjoy any time)
Add 1 tablespoon raw cacao powder. Mix with a hand blender until smooth.

VANILLA AGAR PUDDING (enjoy any time)
Add 1 teaspoon vanilla extract. Mix with a hand blender until smooth.

LEMON CUSTARD AGAR PUDDING (enjoy any time)
Add the grated peel of 1 lemon. Mix with a hand blender until smooth.

PEANUT BUTTER CUP AGAR PUDDING (This will count as your MUFA, but it's so worth it!)
Add 1 tablespoon natural peanut butter to Chocolate Mousse Agar Pudding. Mix with a hand blender until smooth.

BERRY MOUSSE AGAR PUDDING (count as 1 high-hydro fruit)
Add 1 cup mixed berries. Mix with a hand blender until smooth.

*This is on the freebie list in Chapter 6 (page 106) so if you want seconds—go for it!

GOOD DECISIONS CACAO CHIA PUDDING*

MAKES 4 SERVINGS

This is so easy to make and considered just a hydro-booster (unless you add a high-hydro fruit). It's a great way to satisfy a sweet craving and stay full at the same time.

½ cup chia seeds
1 cup unsweetened almond milk
2 teaspoons raw cacao powder
1–2 packets stevia

Place the chia seeds in a large bowl.

In a medium bowl, mix together the almond milk, cacao powder, and 1 stevia packet. Add the other packet if not sweet enough.

Pour over the chia seeds and mix well. Let sit for at least 10 minutes.

Mix again and serve.

GOOD DECISIONS VANILLA CHIA PUDDING:*

Replace the raw cacao powder with ½ teaspoon vanilla extract.

*This is on the freebie list in Chapter 6 (page 106) so if you want seconds—go for it!

FREE FROZEN FRUIT SKEWER*

MAKES 1 SERVING

This snack is on the HD freebies list on page 106. As for the grapes, they're the only HD-friendly fruit you can have throughout all the phases—in this skewered, 10-at-a-time form, that is. You can also just freeze the same amount of fruit without the skewers and munch on it for a guilt-free sweet treat (especially for those nighttime snack attacks), but the skewers make this freebie more fun!

10 grapes

10 raspberries

10 blueberries

On 2 wooden skewers, alternately thread the grapes, raspberries, and blueberries.

Freeze for at least 3 hours for an HD lollipop-like snack.

*This is on the freebie list in Chapter 6 (page 106) so if you want seconds—go for it!

NUTMEG PUMPKIN MASH WITH WALNUTS

MAKES 1 SERVING

- ½ can pumpkin puree
- 4 tablespoons Chia Gel (page 158)
- ½ teaspoon vanilla extract
- ½ teaspoon ground nutmeg
- 1 packet stevia
- 6 walnut halves

In a medium bowl, combine the pumpkin, gel, vanilla, nutmeg, and stevia. Pour into a 6-ounce ramekin lightly coated with cooking spray. Microwave on high power for 2 minutes, or until cooked through (and no longer wet in the middle).

Top with the walnuts.

CHIA SMOOTHIE

MAKES 1 SERVING

You may add 1 packet of stevia or Truvia to add sweetness (though many times this is not necessary!). Experiment with different fruits, too. This smoothie is delicious, filling, and packed with so many nutrients!

1 cup fresh or frozen berries, sliced peach, or cubed mango

½ cup unsweetened almond milk

½ cup water

1 tablespoon chia seeds or 3 tablespoons Chia Gel (page 158)

3 ice cubes

In a blender, combine the fruit, almond milk, water, chia seeds or gel, and ice cubes. Blend until smooth.

JICAMA-NUT SANDWICH

MAKES 1 SERVING

This is a great way to eat nut butter if you want it as your HD-friendly MUFA option for the day. Jicama is crunchy and can be cut into circular slices that make for a healthy canvas for nut butters. Just be careful to not cut the jicama slices too thin or they will break. Save the leftover sliced jicama for additional nut sandwiches, or add it to other HD dishes.

2 slices jicama, peeled and cut into thin circular slices

1 tablespoon natural peanut butter or almond butter, or 2 tablespoons chia peanut butter or chia almond butter (see note)

On 1 slice of the jicama, spread the nut butter or chia nut butter. Top with another slice to make a sandwich.

Note: Simply add 1 tablespoon Chia Gel (page 158) to 1 tablespoon nut butter for a "hydro-stretch."

KALE CHIPS*

MAKES 2 SERVINGS

Kale chips seem to be very popular nowadays. You can buy them at many health food stores. (I even saw a box at my local gas station.) The thing is, they are easy to make at home, and this way you are in control of the ingredients, especially the oil! Serve with HD yogurt dips or high-hydro bean dips.

1 bunch kale (curly or dinosaur), stems removed and cut into 3-inch pieces (see note)

Seasonings of choice to taste (garlic powder, onion powder, kelp powder, or nutritional yeast are good decisions)

Preheat the oven to 350°F. Line a baking sheet with parchment paper.

Place kale pieces on the baking sheet. Lightly coat with cooking spray and season to taste. Bake for 15 minutes, or until the edges are brown.

Note: I recommend using kitchen scissors to cut the kale. Also, make sure the kale is totally dry so it won't be soggy.

*This is on the freebie list in Chapter 6 (page 106) so if you want seconds—go for it!

NORI VEGETABLE WRAP*

MAKES 1 SERVING

This is a freebie snack to enjoy any time you feel like having something to eat. It is easy to grab on the go. I always have a few in my fridge. It's fun to cut them in 1-inch circles to look like sushi, but you can eat them whole or halved. You decide.

1 zucchini, cut into matchsticks

1 carrot, cut into matchsticks

Handful of shredded cabbage

1 sheet nori

2 tablespoons Good Decisions Dressing (pages 189 to 192; the miso one is great) or unlimited condiment (page 82; rice wine vinegar is also great)

Place the zucchini, carrots, and cabbage in the center of the nori. Coat with the dressing or condiment and roll. Use a little water to seal, if needed. Refrigerate for a couple of minutes to harden.

NORI VEGETABLE HUMMUS WRAP:

Spread ¼ cup hummus on the nori before stuffing.

*This is on the freebie list in Chapter 6 (page 106) so if you want seconds—go for it!

ROASTED CHIA NORI STRIPS*

MAKES 2 SERVINGS

I add chia seeds to this delicious, crunchy snack for a hydro-boost. However, you can eliminate the chia seeds if you want them plain.

10 sheets nori

2 tablespoons chia seeds

Preheat the oven to 275°F. Line a baking sheet with parchment paper.

Lay out the nori shiny side down. Lightly coat with olive oil spray and fold once. Cut each sheet into 4 or 5 strips and place on the baking sheet. Coat lightly with cooking spray and sprinkle with the chia seeds.

Bake for 10 minutes, or until crispy. Cool on a rack for 15 minutes.

Note: The strips can be stored in an airtight container for up to 1 week.

*This is on the freebie list in Chapter 6 (page 106) so if you want seconds—go for it!

DIFFERENT WAYS TO MAKE HD POPCORN

MAKES 1 SERVING

The microwave popcorn you buy at the store often has a long ingredient list that can be hard to decipher. Microwave your own "naked" popcorn instead. Then dress it up on your terms.

2 tablespoons kernel popcorn

Put the kernels in a brown paper bag, fold over the top two times, and microwave on high power for 2½ minutes, or until popping stops.

You can use a number of seasonings to dress up your popcorn. Here are a few of my favorites.

SEAWEED POPCORN

Crumble 10 toasted nori strips (2 sheets) in the bag and mix thoroughly. You can use your own strips (page 228) or store-brought varieties.

CINNAMON POPCORN

Lightly coat with cooking spray (just enough so the ingredients stick). Add stevia and cinnamon to taste and mix thoroughly. This is a sweet, crunchy treat.

GARLIC POPCORN

Lightly coat with cooking spray. Add ½ teaspoon each kelp powder, nutritional yeast, and garlic powder and mix thoroughly.

AVOCADO EGGS

MAKES 1 SERVING

This is like a deviled eggs recipe without the mayo. I use 1 yolk per serving and it's a real treat. These eggs are a good way to get your HD-friendly MUFA in, with ¼ avocado.

- 3 hard-cooked eggs, peeled and halved lengthwise
- ¼ avocado
- 2 tablespoons lemon juice
- ½ teaspoon onion powder
- Dash of dried cilantro

Remove the egg yolks and place only 1 in a medium bowl. Arrange the egg whites on a small plate.

Add the avocado to the yolk and mix until creamy. Mix in the lemon juice, onion powder, and cilantro.

Spoon the mixture evenly into the egg white halves.

ROASTED CHICKPEAS

MAKES 4 SERVINGS

This is a delicious, crunchy, high-hydro protein snack! Pair these chickpeas with some HD Crudité (page 165) on the run.

- 1 can (14–19 ounces) no-salt-added chickpeas, rinsed and drained (see note on page 183)
- ½ teaspoon garlic powder
- ½ teaspoon paprika

Preheat the oven to 400°F. Line a baking sheet with foil.

In a large bowl, add the chickpeas, garlic powder, and paprika and mix together until evenly coated.

Spread the chickpeas on the baking sheet. Bake for 1 hour, stirring occasionally, or until the chickpeas are hard and crunchy.

POACHED CINNAMON PEARS

MAKES 4 SERVINGS

4 pears

1 cinnamon stick

1 teaspoon vanilla extract

1 teaspoon grated lemon peel

2 packets stevia

6 walnut halves (optional)

Place the pears in a large pot. Fill with water so the pears are covered. Add the cinnamon stick, vanilla, lemon peel, and stevia.

Bring to a boil and cook for 15 to 20 minutes, or until soft.

Remove the pears and allow to cool for 10 minutes. Cut in half and sprinkle evenly with the walnuts, if using.

RASPBERRY-CACAO SORBET

MAKES 1 SERVING

You can use any frozen berries you want for this very easy sorbet.

1 cup frozen raspberries

¼ cup unsweetened almond milk

1 cup ice

2 teaspoons raw cacao powder

1 tablespoon chia seeds (optional)

1–2 packets stevia

In a blender, combine the raspberries, almond milk, ice, cacao powder, chia seeds (if using), and stevia to taste. Blend until smooth.

CLARA, 52, *Lost 30 Pounds*

Before HD: My husband, Steve, started the HD plan a month before I did, and I quickly witnessed infectious changes in his mood and energy. I considered myself educated about good nutrition, and I've even used food to heal myself from medical illnesses. But when I hit my midforties, I began to suffer from physical pain that only medicine could alleviate—and only mildly. So I was just getting through one day at a time and gaining weight as a result. This continued until my early fifties. Then, while on vacation in July 2013, I started to follow what my husband was doing when we were dining out; his new approach to eating was simple, mindful, and practical. I returned home 3 pounds thinner than when I left, and I felt better, too. I knew then that I needed to meet Keren and get to know the HD plan better.

Starting strong: Within minutes of meeting Keren, I knew that her practical approach to making good nutritional choices would work (despite any medical issues I was having). Starting strong meant logging what I ate; when I ate; and how I felt before, during, and after I ate. As she suggested, becoming aware of my patterns was critical to my success. Logging into my notes app on my smartphone became my new habit. It kept me accountable and aware, and I began to notice how little changes made big differences.

New foods: Chia, chia, chia! I had heard of chia seeds prior to the HD plan but had never used them. Now I know firsthand the amazing benefits of these seeds for improved health. Chia Gel doubles the volume of what you're eating, which is essential in the beginning of a weight-loss program. If you are used to overeating, you'll appreciate how chia adds bulk to snacks and meals. Overall, finding new ways to prepare food with chia has been fun.

Unexpected bonus: Everything about the HD plan is a bonus! It is a practical, clean way to eat whole foods, regardless of food preferences or restrictions. The fact that there are no crazy shakes, no vitamin marketing, and no calorie counting are also great bonuses. It is just a real-life approach to health, minus the fads. And my inflammation disappeared, which was more than a bonus; it helped me finally get my life back. Now I can do a 40-minute, high-impact workout on the elliptical trainer. I can also go on quick-paced walks again.

Lesson learned: Be mindful, be aware, and make good decisions about your nutrition. I now see the old you-are-what-you-eat mantra as "you feel what you eat!" And because of HD, I feel good. My favorite lesson: If you model behaviors instead of just preaching them, the people around you begin to change. Now that my husband and I are walking the walk (instead of just talking the talk), our kids have started following the HD plan, too, and they have seen tremendous benefits. I often hear my daughter joke around and say, "Chia is life!" Or I'll hear my son say, "I still have one carbohydrate left today; this is how I plan to use it." We each have our own approach as to what works best, but we share recipes and little tricks we come up with along the way. We also exercise together when we have the chance.

New mantra: Patterns, patterns, choices, choices, decisions, decisions.

Sustaining in HD: Sustaining anything in life means not becoming obsessed. If I go to a party, banquet, or wedding and indulge in non-HD-friendly foods, I don't feel guilty. I just go back to my healthy patterns the next meal. It's all a choice!

Never misses: Bad carbohydrates and sugar. I no longer fall into the carb-sugar "coma."

Inspiring words: I am a 52-year-old woman who feels like a teenager again (but a wise one this time). My husband feels young again, too. Our entire family (including our daughter and son) is down 130 pounds! We are having the time of our lives, and we can sustain the HD plan even when out and about or faced with a challenging day. We no longer use food negatively to deal with life; we use it positively to make life better!

AFTERWORD

The experiences I have had with my clients are invaluable. They have taught me that making the very important decision to take control of your health and your body is connected to living your life at a higher state of focus—in HD. People from so many different backgrounds have walked through the doors of Decision Nutrition, and I have witnessed their personal voyages unfold before me. The time they spent with me resulted in not only weight loss but also new beginnings.

As many of my clients have discovered (and shared with you in this book), making the *decision* to live in HD brings a wealth of benefits. Besides weight loss and healthy vitality, you get a huge boost of confidence from knowing you made a *decision* and that you followed it through to success. People have emerged from their HD journeys more focused on their families, their friendships, their lifelong dreams and careers.

You may have picked up this book because you needed to lose the extra weight on your body, but I guarantee that as the pounds come off, you will gain a new perspective on your life. There's nothing superficial about a life that is more clear and focused than you ever imagined.

What can *you* accomplish when you live in HD? Only you can decide. I wish you the joy of living decisively!

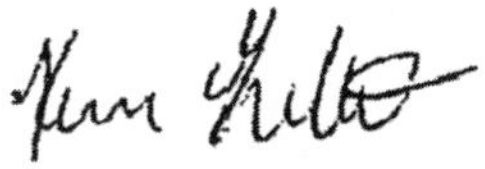

Keren Gilbert, MS, RD

APPENDIX A
MY HD CONTRACT
to Live Decisively to Improve My Health and My Body

(ALSO AVAILABLE AT DECISIONNUTRITION.COM)

What is it that you want from your HD experience? Write down what you desire to achieve. Not the weight loss per se, but the life changes you anticipate as a result. What are your ultimate goals?

Write down affirmatively what it will feel like when you have achieved all of your goals. Be specific and write in the present tense. Remember: Your written words are a powerful tool to help strengthen your intentions and turn your thoughts into reality.

What daily decisions can you start making to achieve your goals? Think about the daily habits that are hindering your weight loss. Decide now how you can replace them with new ones. This is just a start to increase your awareness of your own habits.

1.

2.

3.

I, ______________________ , understand that my decisions up to this point
(name)
have interfered with me attaining the goals I want for myself and I am ready to change my life.

Initial these:

- [ ] I will read over my goals and my decisions daily.
- [ ] I will make the changes necessary to achieve all my health and body aspirations.
- [ ] I will be honest with myself about the decisions I make.
- [ ] I will log my food choices every day.

I am ready to make this commitment to myself starting today ______________
(today's date)

and on ____________________ weigh ________
(pick a date 12 weeks from today)

It is done.

____

Signature Date

APPENDIX B
HD FOOD LOG

Name

Date

Refer to the Hunger Determination Scale on page 29 to see what number you relate to before and after snacks/meals.

MEAL	TIME	FOOD & DRINK DECISIONS	
BREAKFAST	HD Scale before: HD Scale after:		
SNACK			
LUNCH			
SNACK			
DINNER			
SNACK			

	NOTES (HEALTH DERAILERS / GOOD DECISIONS)

APPENDIX C WEEKLY GOAL TRACKER

THIS WEEK'S GOALS

I will accomplish the above goals this week.

Signature Date

APPENDIX D NAVIGATING THE SUPERMARKET

ICONS

☺	HIGH-HYDRO
*	HD-FRIENDLY
**	HIGH-HYDRO CARBOHYDRATE
†	HIGH-HYDRO PROTEIN
♥	MUFA

Since the HD plan focuses on high-hydro vegetables and fruits, try to always start out in the produce section of the supermarket to fill your cart with all of your favorites!

FRESH VEGETABLES

Within the produce section, there are high-hydro vegetables that I want you to focus on, HD-friendly vegetables you can mix with high-hydro vegetables, and vegetables that are considered high-hydro carbohydrates. Each one is classified here.

FYI: Many times vegetables are precut into ready-to-buy platters. I know that this can be costly, but it's a convenient way to get some raw high-hydro vegetables in your diet. This can be a great option to put in your cart. A beautiful vegetable platter doesn't only have to be for guests!

○ Acorn squash**
○ Artichokes☺
○ Arugula*
○ Asparagus☺
○ Bean sprouts☺
○ Beets☺
○ Bell peppers (all kinds)☺
○ Broccoli☺
○ Broccoli rabe☺
○ Brussels sprouts☺
○ Butternut squash**
○ Cabbage☺

- ○ Carrots☺
- ○ Celery *
- ○ Collard greens☺
- ○ Cucumber*
- ○ Dandelion greens☺
- ○ Eggplant*
- ○ Endive*
- ○ Escarole*
- ○ Jicama☺
- ○ Jerusalem artichoke☺
- ○ Kale☺
- ○ Kohlrabi☺
- ○ Mustard greens☺
- ○ Mushrooms*
- ○ Okra☺
- ○ Onions☺
- ○ Parsnips**
- ○ Peas†
- ○ Snow peas☺
- ○ Spaghetti squash☺
- ○ Spinach☺
- ○ Sweet potato**
- ○ Swiss chard☺
- ○ Tomatoes*
- ○ Turnips☺
- ○ Yellow squash☺
- ○ Zucchini☺

FRESH FRUIT

Again, begin to see all the fruits in terms of high-hydro and HD-friendly. I encourage you to stock up on the high-hydro fruits especially in Start Strong phase. Then you can add an HD-friendly fruit as you progress into Still Focused.

FYI: Always look for fruits that are in season. Remember that grapes are an HD-friendly fruit, but 10 frozen grapes are allowed in the Start Strong phase, so throw them in your cart and make frozen fruit skewers!

- ○ Apples☺
- ○ Apricots☺
- ○ Avocados ♥
- ○ Banana*
- ○ Blackberries☺
- ○ Blueberries☺
- ○ Cantaloupe*
- ○ Cherries*
- ○ Clementines☺
- ○ Cranberries☺
- ○ Figs, fresh☺
- ○ Grapes*
- ○ Grapefruit☺
- ○ Honeydew

- ○ Lemons☺
- ○ Limes☺
- ○ Mango☺
- ○ Kiwifruit☺
- ○ Oranges☺
- ○ Papaya☺
- ○ Peaches☺
- ○ Pears☺
- ○ Pineapples*
- ○ Plums☺
- ○ Pomegranate seeds☺
- ○ Pumpkin☺
- ○ Raspberries☺
- ○ Strawberries☺
- ○ Watermelon*

DAIRY

FYI: Shirataki noodles and kelp noodles are most often found in the dairy section, not the pasta section, as they are refrigerated. Kelp noodles may be harder to find. They can also be found in the Asian or international foods aisle. I include egg subsitutes to have on hand for those busy mornings.

- ○ Egg substitutes*–I like Papetti's All White 100% Liquid Egg Whites or Eggology 100% Egg Whites
- ○ Eggs*
- ○ Greek yogurt, plain (like Fage or Chobani)*
- ○ Hummus (Tribe, Sabra, Good Neighbors)☺
- ○ Kelp noodles☺
- ○ Shirataki noodles (different shapes)☺
- ○ Tofu (firm, extra-firm)*
- ○ Unsweetened almond milk (40 calories cup or less, like Almond Breeze)
- ○ Unsweetened vanilla almond milk (40 calories cup or less, like Almond Breeze)

FROZEN FOODS AISLE

I encourage my clients to stock up on frozen vegetables. There is nothing wrong with preparing frozen veggies—they're often flash frozen, which preserves the nutrients, and can be a lot easier on your wallet. As long as they are plain with no sugar or salt added, you are good to go. I have listed my favorite go-to frozen high-hydro vegetables and high-hydro fruits here.

FYI: Frozen fruits are wonderful to keep on-hand for smoothies!

- ○ Artichokes☺
- ○ Asparagus☺
- ○ Bell peppers (green, red, or yellow)☺
- ○ Broccoli☺
- ○ Broccoli rabe☺
- ○ Brussels sprouts☺
- ○ Carrots☺
- ○ Collard greens☺
- ○ Kale☺
- ○ Okra☺
- ○ Peas†
- ○ Snow peas☺
- ○ Spinach☺
- ○ Swiss chard
- ○ Yellow squash☺
- ○ Zucchini☺

- ○ Blackberries☺
- ○ Blueberries☺
- ○ Mango☺
- ○ Peaches☺
- ○ Pears☺
- ○ Raspberries☺
- ○ Strawberries☺

Here are some other foods you can grab while you're in the freezer section.

- ○ Amy's California Burger (light in sodium)
- ○ Gardenburger Black Bean Chipotle
- ○ Salmon fillets*
- ○ Shrimp*
- ○ Veggie burgers (I like Dr. Praeger's California Veggie Burger)†

CANNED & INTERNATIONAL FOODS

As you explore the canned aisles, remember to look for No-Salt-Added varieties.

- ○ Adzuki beans†
- ○ Black beans†
- ○ Black-eyed peas†
- ○ Chickpeas (garbanzo beans)†
- ○ Dried beans, peas, and lentils (without flavoring packets)†
- ○ Fava beans†
- ○ Great Northern beans†
- ○ Kidney beans†
- ○ Lentils†

- ○ Mung beans †
- ○ Navy beans
- ○ Olives ♥
- ○ Pinto beans†
- ○ Tomatoes—I like Muir Glen Organic or Whole Foods 365*
- ○ White beans†
- ○ Agar☺
- ○ Arame☺
- ○ Dulse☺
- ○ Kombu☺
- ○ Nori☺

BREADS, CEREALS & GRAINS

Explore the aisles for breads, crackers, and wraps that fit the HD-friendly carbohydrate guidelines: 100 calories or less; 3 grams of fiber or more. I listed some brands below but you can do some investigative work and try different brands that fit the HD criteria. Remember, in Start Strong to limit carbs to 2 per day with at least 1 from the high-hydro carbohydrate** option.

Try to find cereals that fall under the HD-friendly carbohydrate guidelines: 150 calories or less; 5 grams of fiber or more. Watch the sugar grams in your cereal! Look for 6 grams of sugar or less per serving.

FYI: You can order Decision Nutrition Chia Bagels at decisionnutrition.com or amazon.com.

- ○ Amaranth**
- ○ Barbara's Original Puffins cereal
- ○ Barley**
- ○ Brown rice**
- ○ Buckwheat**
- ○ Decision Nutrition Chia Bagels*
- ○ Decision Nutrition Chia Chips*
- ○ Farro**
- ○ FiberRich Bran Crackers*
- ○ Food for Life Ezekiel 4:9*
- ○ Kashi Heart to Heart Cereal*
- ○ La Tortilla Factory Low Carb Tortillas*
- ○ McCann's Oatmeal
- ○ Popcorn*
- ○ Quaker Oatmeal
- ○ Quinoa**
- ○ Rye berries**
- ○ Ryvita Dark Rye Crispbread*
- ○ Tumaro's Low in Carbs Multi-Grain Tortillas*
- ○ Uncle Sam Oatmeal
- ○ Wasa Fiber Rye Crispbread*

POULTRY & FISH

The best advice is to buy your poultry and fish from reputable markets. For poultry, always look that it is USDA certified organic.

- ○ Chicken, ground (extra lean)*
- ○ Chicken breast (skin off)*
- ○ Cod*
- ○ Crab*
- ○ Flounder*
- ○ Halibut*
- ○ Orange roughy*
- ○ Salmon, wild (canned in water or fresh)*
- ○ Scallops*
- ○ Shrimp*
- ○ Tuna (canned in water or fresh)*
- ○ Turkey, ground (at least 93% lean)*
- ○ Turkey breast (skin off)*

NUTS & SEEDS

You can now find nuts in individual packs to make portioning easier.

- ○ Almond butter ♥
- ○ Almonds ♥
- ○ Chia seeds (hydro-boosters!!)
- ○ Peanut butter, natural ♥
- ○ Pistachios ♥
- ○ Pumpkin seeds, unsalted ♥
- ○ Sunflower seeds, unsalted ♥
- ○ Walnuts ♥

CONDIMENTS/MISCELLANEOUS

Always have the following condiments/miscellaneous items stocked in your kitchen. I've included suggested brands for each.

- ○ Bragg Liquid Aminos
- ○ Cacao powder (Navitas Natural)
- ○ Cooking sprays (Spectrum)
- ○ Dandelion tea (Alvita, Celebration Herbals)
- ○ Herbs and spices
- ○ Horseradish (Silver Spring Foods, Annie's)
- ○ Hot-pepper sauce
- ○ Miso paste (Maruman, Hikari Organic, Eden Foods)

- Mustard (Annie's, Eden Foods)
- Nettle tea (Alvita, Celebration Herbals)
- Pasta sauce (Rao's, San Marzano)
- Salsa (Green Mountain Gringo, Muir Glen, Amy's)
- Seltzer (La Croix, San Pellegrino, Perrier)
- Stevia (NuNaturals, Sweet Leaf, Truvia)
- Tamari, low sodium (San-J, Eden Foods)
- True lemon/true lime packets
- Vinegars (Bionatural, Bragg, Spectrum)

SNACKS

Most of the foods on the 12-week plan are fresh and whole and always ready to grab and go out the door like all raw veggies from the HD Crudité or all the high-hydro fruits on page 72. But I understand that there are times you just need a grab and go item that you can keep in your pantry, suitcase (when travelling), car, bag, gym locker etc. Here are some of my favorites. Always check decisionnutrition.com for updated lists. I am always on the hunt for new grab and gos!

Nutrition Bars

- Kind Bars with 6 grams of sugar or less (MUFA)–Madagascar Vanilla Almond, Caramel Almond & Sea Salt, Dark Chocolate Nuts & Sea Salt, Dark Chocolate Mocha Almond, Roasted Jalapeño
- FiberLoveBars by Gnu Foods (HD-Friendly Carb)
- Healthy Warrior Chia Bars (HD-Friendly Carb)–Chocolate Peanut Butter is the best!

High-Hydro Dried Fruits

- Matt's Munchies–Island Mango, Mango, Applelicious, Tangy Apricot
- FruitChia Bars
- Made in Nature Figs, Plums and Apricots
- Just Tomatoes Just Strawberries, or Just Mango
- Nature's All Organic Strawberries
- Bare Fruit Organic Granny Smith Apple Chips, Gluten-Free

High-Hydro Proteins

- Cruncha ma-me freeze-dried edamame snacks, Naked or Lightly Seasoned
- The Good Bean Crispy Crunchy Chickpeas Sea Salt Flavor
- Wild Garden Hummus Dip single serve packages
- Sabra Hummus single serving packages
- Just Tomatoes Just Peas

MUFAS

- Wonderful Roasted & Salted Pistachios
- Blue Diamond Almonds Grab & Go Bags, 100 calories per bag
- Justin's All-Natural Classic Almond Butter or Peanut Butter 1.15 oz. packs

Seaweeds

- SeaSnax Roasted Seaweed Snacks, Grab & Go packs
- Annie Chun's Roasted Seaweed Snacks

HD-Friendly Chips and Crackers

- The Mediterranean Snack Company Baked Lentil Chips, 22 chips
- Mary's Gone Crackers (gluten-free)
- Beanitos Original Black Bean Chips with Sea Salt, 13 chips
- Suzie's Thin Cakes Corn, Quinoa & Sesame (gluten-free)–4.6 oz
- Wasa Crispbread
- Fiber Rich Crispbread

Yogurts—HD-Friendly Proteins

- Fage 0%
- Siggi's 0%

ENDNOTES

CHAPTER 1

1 Wansink, B., and J. Sobal. Mindless eating: The 200 daily food decisions we overlook. *Environment and Behavior* 39, no. 1 (January 2007): 106–23.

2 Burkitt, D. P. Some diseases characteristic of modern Western civilization. *British Medical Journal* 1 (February 1973): 274–78.

3 Andon, M. B., and J. W. Anderson. The oatmeal-cholesterol connection: 10 years later. *American Journal of Lifestyle Medicine* 2, no. 1 (January/February 2008): 51–57.

4 Bazzano, L. A., J. He, L. G. Ogden, C. Loria, S. Vupputuri, L. Myers, and P. K. Whelton. Legume consumption and risk of coronary heart disease in US men and women. *Archives of Internal Medicine* 161, no. 21 (November 2001): 2573–78.

5 Maeda, H., R. Yamamoto, K. Hirao, and O. Tochikubo. Effects of agar (kanten) diet on obese patients with impaired glucose tolerance and type 2 diabetes. *Diabetes, Obesity and Metabolism* 7, no. 1 (January 2005): 40–46.

CHAPTER 6

1 Epstein, L. H., K. A. Carr, M. D. Cavanaugh, R. A. Paluch, and M. E. Bouton. Long-term habituation to food in obese and nonobese women. *American Journal of Clinical Nutrition* 94, no. 2 (August 2011): 371–76.

CHAPTER 7

1 Blundell, J. E., and A. J. Hill. Paradoxical effects of an intense sweetener (aspartame) on appetite. *Lancet* 327, no. 8489 (May 1986): 1092–93.

2 Rogers, P. J., J. A. Carlyle, A. J. Hill, and J. E. Blundell. Uncoupling sweet taste and calories: Comparison of the effects of glucose and three intense sweeteners on hunger and food intake. *Physiology & Behavior* 43, no. 5 (1988): 547–52.

3 Yang, Q. Gain Weight by "going diet"? Artificial sweeteners and the neurobiology of sugar cravings. *Yale Journal of Biology and Medicine* (June 2010).

4 Pan, A., Q. Sun, A. M. Bernstein, M. B. Schulze, J. E. Manson, M. J. Stampfer, W. C. Willett, and F. B. Hu. Red meat consumption and mortality: results from 2 prospective cohort studies. *Archives of Internal Medicine* 172, no. 7 (April 2012):555–63. doi: 10.1001/archinternmed.2011.2287. Epub 2012 Mar 12.

5 Pan, A., Q. Sun, A. M. Bernstein, M. B. Schulze, J. E. Manson, W. C. Willett, and F. B. Hu. Red meat consumption and risk of type 2 diabetes: 3 cohorts of US adults and an updated meta-analysis. *American Journal of Clinical Nutrition.* 94, no. 4 (October 2011):1088–96. doi: 10.3945/ajcn.111.018978. Epub 2011 Aug 10

CHAPTER 8

1 Felman, H. A. Erectile dysfunction and coronary risk factors: prospective results from the Massachusetts male aging study. New England Research Institutes, Watertown, Massachusetts, 02472, USA. *Preventive Medicine* (Impact Factor: 3.5). 04/2000; 30(4):328-38. DOI: 10.1006/pmed.2000.0643.

2 Edward O. Laumann, PhD; Anthony Paik, MA; Raymond C. Rosen, PhD, Sexual dysfunction in the United States: Prevalence and predictors author affiliations: department of sociology, University of Chicago, Chicago, Ill (Dr. Laumann and Mr. Paik); and department of psychiatry, University of Medicine and Denistry of New Jersey—Robert Wood Johnson Medical School, Piscataway (Dr. Rosen). *JAMA.* 1999;281(6):537–44. doi:10.1001/jama.281.6.537.

INDEX

Underscored page references indicate sidebars and tables. **Boldface** references indicate illustrations.

Acorn squash
  Bean-Stuffed Acorn Squash, 206
Action, in Stages of Change model, 24
Agar, 16–17, 80
  Agar Pudding, 220
Aging, weight loss and, 150, 151–52
Alcohol, 38, 111–13, 138, 148–49
Allergies, food, 131–32, 133, 135, 154
Alliums, 81
Almond butter
  Jicama-Nut Sandwich, 225
Almond milk, 84, 116, 135
Aloe vera juice, for digestion, 138
Apples, 8
  Apple-Cinnamon Oatmeal, 172
Arame, 80, 81
  Arame and Kale Salad, 186
Artichokes
  Asparagus and Artichoke Salad, 187
Artificial sweeteners, 35, 82, 113–14, 142
Asparagus
  Asparagus and Artichoke Salad, 187
Avocado
  Avocado Eggs, 230

"**B**aby" excuse, for avoiding HD living, 149
Balsamic vinegar
  Balsamic Chicken, 207
  Balsamic Mustard Dressing, 189
Barley, 14
  Barley Breakfast, 175
Bars, meal-replacement, 154
Beans
  Bean-Stuffed Acorn Squash, 206
  dried, cooking, 159–60
  as high-hydrophilic food, 15, 75–76
  Turkey Chili, 199
  White Bean Dip, 184
Berries. *See also* Raspberries
  Berry Mousse Agar Pudding, 220
  Berry Parfait, 219
  Free Frozen Fruit Skewer, 222
Binge eating, 35–36, 126
Block foods, 12, 14, 142
Blood sugar
  controlling, 7, 8, 17, 73, 78, 113, 121, 136, 140
  negative effects on, 120, 121, 124
Blueberries
  Free Frozen Fruit Skewer, 222
Bread
  choosing, 77, 247
  gluten-free, 134–35
  white, as infrequent food, 124
Breakfast
  Apple-Cinnamon Oatmeal, 172
  Barley Breakfast, 175
  Brussels Egg Scramble, 176
  Chia-Oat Pancake, 177
  Eggsellent Omelet, 178
  Microwave Chia Egg Soufflé, 179
  Quick Cacao Chia Oatmeal, 173
  Quick Chia Oatmeal, 173
  skipping, 30
  Swiss Chard Mini Frittatas, 180
  Tofu Scrambler, 181
  While-You-Sleep Chia Oatmeal, 174
Broccoli
  Broccoli-Red Cabbage Slaw, 188
  Broccoli Soup, 193
  Vegetable-Chia Miso Soup, 198
Brussels sprouts
  Brussels Egg Scramble, 176
  how to cook, 15
  as hydrophilic food, 14–15
Burgers
  Spinach Turkey Burgers, 218
Busy Mama diet character, 36–37, 44, 53, 53–54, 58, 103–5
Butter, as infrequent food, 114–15
B vitamins, 137

Cabbage
  Broccoli-Red Cabbage Slaw, 188
  Cabbage Spaghetti with Ground Chicken, 210
  Nori Vegetable Wrap, 227
Cacao powder
  Chia Cacao Yogurt, 219
  Chocolate Mousse Agar Pudding, 220
  Good Decisions Cacao Chia Pudding, 221
  Quick Cacao Chia Oatmeal, 173
  Raspberry-Cacao Sorbet, 233
Calcium, food sources of, 117
Cancer, 5, 13, 15, 140
Canned foods, choosing, 246–47
Carb fake-out foods, 17, 93
Carbohydrates
  counting, 95
  HD-friendly, 77–78, 247
  high-hydrophilic, 76–77, 134, 169

Carrots
Nori Vegetable Wrap, 227
Vegetable-Chia Miso Soup, 198
Casein, in dairy products, 115, 116
Celiac disease, 133, 134
Cereals
choosing, 247
gluten-free, 134–35
HD-friendly, 77
"Cheat Sheet" plate, for portion control, 89–90, **90**, 92, 107, 119, 171
Cheese, as infrequent food, 116–17
Chia Gel
Balsamic Mustard Dressing, 189
how to make, 11, 158
Lemon-Oregano Dressing, 190
Miso Dressing, 191
Salsa Dressing, 192
storing, 100, 101
uses for, 10, 66, 74, 79, 157–58, 189, 234
Vegetable-Chia Miso Soup, 198
Chia nut butter, 183
Chia seeds. *See also* Chia Gel
benefits of, 11, 138
Chia Cacao Yogurt, 219
Chia-Crusted Salmon, 212
Chia-Oat Pancake, 177
Chia-Raspberry Smash, 185
Chia Smoothie, 224
Good Decisions Cacao Chia Pudding, 221
Good Decisions Vanilla Chia Pudding, 221
as hydro-booster, 9–11, 66, 74, 134
Microwave Chia Egg Soufflé, 179
Quick Cacao Chia Oatmeal, 173
Quick Chia Oatmeal, 173
Roasted Chia Nori Strips, 228
uses for, 10
While-You-Sleep Chia Oatmeal, 174
Chicken
Balsamic Chicken, 207
Cabbage Spaghetti with Ground Chicken, 210
choosing, 248
Cinnamon Chicken, 208
Lemon Grilled Chicken, 209
Chickpeas, 15–16
Chickpea Spread, 183
Roasted Chickpeas, 231
Chili
Turkey Chili, 199
Chips
Kale Chips, 226
Chocolate substitute. *See* Cacao powder
Cholesterol levels
factors improving, 5, 8, 12, 78, 140
fats increasing, 114, 115
high, HD plan approriate for, 136
Chubby Perpetual Exerciser diet character, 33–35, 49, 49–50, 60
Cinnamon
Apple-Cinnamon Oatmeal, 172
Cinnamon Chicken, 208
Cinnamon Popcorn, 229
Poached Cinnamon Pears, 232
Cleanses, juice, 139
Coconut products, 135
Coenzyme Q10, 137
Coffee, 84
Comparisons with others, as form of excusitis, 153
Condiments, 82, 135, 167, 248
Constant Socializer diet character, 37–38, 55, 55
Contemplation, in Stages of Change model, 24
Contract, My HD, 45, 56, 59, 238–39
Cooking spray, 83, 171
Coronary heart disease, 16. *See also* Heart disease
Cravings, 7, 17, 113, 121
Crudité, HD, 165–66

Dairy foods, 115–16, 245
Dairy-free lifestyle, 135
Decision making. *See also* Food decisions
excusitis affecting, 145
in HD living, 237
for weight loss and maintenance, 23, 25, 65
Decision Nutrition Chia Bagels, 26, 78, 247
Decision Nutrition Chia Chips, 78, 126, 168, 247
Detoxification, 67, 84, 139
Diabetes, 8, 17, 78, 120, 121, 136, 140
Diet characters
The Busy Mama, 36–37, 44, 53, 53–54, 58, 103–5
Chubby Perpetual Exerciser, 33–35, 49, 49–50, 60
The Constant Socializer, 37–38, 55, 55
The Enormous Iron Man, 38–39, 45, 59
On-the-Go Gobbler, 32–33, 44, 47, 47–48, 57
The Plump Know-It-All, 35–36, 51, 51–52
Digestive enzymes, 138
Digestive health, improving, 8, 138
Dijon mustard
Balsamic Mustard Dressing, 189
Dill
Dill Yogurt Dip, 182
Dips and spreads
Black Bean Dip, 184
Chia-Raspberry Smash, 185
Chickpea Spread, 183
Edamame Dip, 185
White Bean Dip, 184
Yogurt Dip, 182
Diseases, effect of diet on, 4–5
Dried fruits, 74
Dulse, 80

Eating out. *See* Restaurant meals
Eating plan, HD. *See* HD eating plan

Edamame
Edamame Dip, 185
Eggplant
HD Ratatouille, 200
Eggs
Avocado Eggs, 230
Brussels Egg Scramble, 176
Eggsellent Omelet, 178
Microwave Chia Egg Soufflé, 179
Swiss Chard Mini Frittatas, 180
Energy bars, 36
Enormous Iron Man diet character, 38–39, 45, 59
Entrées
Baked Tofu, 216
Balsamic Chicken, 207
Bean-Stuffed Acorn Squash, 206
Cabbage Spaghetti with Ground Chicken, 210
Chia-Crusted Salmon, 212
Cinnamon Chicken, 208
Easy Fish, 211
HD Tuna Salad, 215
Lemon Grilled Chicken, 209
Rosemary-Lemon Salmon, 213
Salmon Salad Nori Wrap, 214
Scallop Stir-Fry Shirataki, 217
Spinach Turkey Burgers, 218
Excusitis, 145–53
Exercise, 139–41, 149

Fast food, 5, 33
Fats, dietary
HD-friendly, 78–79
unhealthy, 114–15, 119, 136
Fat storage, causes of, 30
Fiber
health benefits of, 5, 6
insoluble, 4, 6–7
recommended vs. actual intake of, 6
soluble, 4, 7–9
Fish
Chia-Crusted Salmon, 212
choosing, 248
Easy Fish, 211
HD Tuna Salad, 215
Rosemary-Lemon Salmon, 213
Salmon Salad Nori Wrap, 214
Flavorings, 82–83
Flour, refined white, 5, 124
Food additives, 118, 118, 120
Food allergies, 131–32, 133, 135, 154
Food as medicine, 3
Food costs, as excuse for unhealthy eating, 150–51
Food decisions. *See also* Decision making
bad, hunger leading to, 30
daily number of, 3–4, 5, 152
pre-HD, analyzing, 27–32
Food intolerances, 132, 133
Food likes and dislikes. *See* Block foods
Food logging
importance of, 45–46, 86, 155, 234
sample of, 55, 55
Food log sheets, 28, 40–41, 46, 240–41
Food shopping, 147, 151, 243–48
Food temptations, as excuse for unhealthy eating, 152–53
Food weaknesses, managing, 148–49
Freebie foods, 106
Freshman 15, preventing, 151
Fried foods, as infrequent foods, 117–18
Frozen foods, choosing, 245–46
Fruits. *See also specific fruits*
choosing, 244–45, 246
Free Frozen Fruit Skewer, 222
HD-friendly, 73–74
high-hydrophilic, 72–73, 121, 134
pectin in, 13, 16
prepping and storing, 101

Garlic powder
Garlic Popcorn, 229
Gazpacho
Gazpacho Soup, 194
Gluten-free foods, 133–35, 154
Gluten intolerance, 132, 134, 154
Goals
analyzing, 238, 239
of diet characters, 32
reaching, 70
weekly, 59–60, 242
writing about, 43–44
Grains
choosing, 247
cooking, 158, 158–59
Grapes
Free Frozen Fruit Skewer, 222
Greek yogurt, 78, 135

Habits, changing
stages for, 23–25, **23**
for weight loss, 238
Hand blender, 100, 167
HD "Cheat Sheet" plate, for portion control, 89–90, **90**, 92, 107, 119, 171
HD eating plan
additional foods in, 80–84
core foods in (*see* HD-friendly foods; High-hydrophilic foods; Hydro-boosters; IFs)
healthy alterations in, 131–41
phases of
Soaring in HD, 69–70
Start Strong (*see* Start Strong phase, of HD eating plan)
Still Focused in HD, 68–69, 110–11, 125
HD Food Log. *See also* Food logging; Food log sheets
HD-friendly foods, 66, 134
carbohydrates, 77–78, 247
fruits, 73–74

liquids, 83–84
MUFA, 78–79
proteins, 76
vegetables, 72
HD-friendly kitchen tools, 100
HD living
benefits of, 237
decisions in, 23, 25
excuses interfering with, 145–53
exercise in, 139–41
juice cleanses unnecessary in, 138–39
reasons for wanting, 43
supplements in, 137–38
writing about goals for, 43–44
HD satiation, 6, 12, 13, 29, 35, 36, 66, 100, 161. *See also* Satiety
HD success stories
Amy, 61
Cheryl, 26
Clara, 234–35
Diane, 86–87
Ilana, 18–19
Liana, 154–55
Liz, 168–69
Lyssa, 142–43
Paul, 42
Randi, 126–27
Steve, 107
Health derailers
common, 40–41, 41
of diet characters, 33–39
methods of identifying, 39–41
Healthy foods, lack of, preventing weight loss, 33
Heart disease, 5, 8, 12, 78, 115, 119, 140
Herbs, 81
High-hydrophilic foods, 65–66, 134
carbohydrates, 76–77, 169
fruits, 72–73, 121
grains, 158, 158–59
health benefits of, 5, 6
properties of, 4
proteins, 75–76, 136, 159–60
seaweed, 80–81
top ten, 9–17
vegetables (*see* Vegetables, high-hydrophilic)
Hippocrates, 3, 4
Horseradish
Horseradish Yogurt Dip, 182
Hummus
Nori Vegetable Hummus Wrap, 227
Hunger
after eating HD-friendly vegetables, 72
foods preventing, 7, 10, 12, 74
ignoring signals of, 33
Hunger Determination Scale, 28, 29, 30–32, 40, 65, 76, 102, 106
Hydration, chia seeds improving, 11
Hydro-boosters, 66, 67, 74, 77
Hydrophilic foods. *See* High-hydrophilic foods

IFs (infrequent foods)
avoiding or controlling, 19, 84–85
complete list of, 110, 111–25
difficulty avoiding, 67
exercise and, 140
thinking about, before eating, 109–10
when to introduce, 66, 110–11
Impotence, exercise preventing, 141
International foods, choosing, 246–47

Jicama
Jicama-Nut Sandwich, 225
Juice cleanses, 138–39
Julienne cutter, 100

Kale
Arame and Kale Salad, 186
Kale Chips, 226
Kanten. *See* Agar
Kelp noodles, 80, 245
Kelp supplements, 138
Keren's reminders, 101–2
Kidney beans, as hydrophilic food, 15
Kitchen tools, HD-friendly, 100
Kombu, 80

Lactose intolerance, 115, 132, 135
Lemons
Lemon Custard Agar Pudding, 220
Lemon Grilled Chicken, 209
Lemon-Oregano Dressing, 190
Rosemary-Lemon Salmon, 213
Lentils
Lentil Soup, 196
Lima beans
Lima Bean-Okra Soup, 197
Liquids, HD-friendly, 83–84

Maintenance, in Stages of Change model, 24
Margarine, as infrequent food, 114–15
Mashing vegetables, 167
Mason jars, 100
Meal planning
for HD plan success, 91, 107, 127
lack of, 35
Meal preparation
guidelines, 36–37
building a wrap, 164–65
cooking beans, 159–60
cooking high-hydro grains, 158, 159–60
cooking vegetables, 166–67
for HD crudité, 165–66
for HD salad, 161–64
making chia gel, 157–58
lack of, 35
Meal-replacement bars, 154
Meal skipping, 30, 33, 36

Meats, red and processed, as infrequent foods, 119–20
Menopause, as excuse for weight-loss difficulty, 151–52
Menstruation, as excuse for poor eating, 148
Menu plan, 14-day Start Strong, 91–92, 92–99
Metabolism
 factors decreasing, 112, 114, 115, 150
 factors increasing, 137–38, 140
Mindless eating, 31–32, 36, 37, 39
Miso paste
 Miso Dressing, 191
 Vegetable-Chia Miso Soup, 198
Monounsaturated fats. *See* MUFAs
Mood, exercise improving, 140
Mucilage, 8–9
MUFAs, as HD-friendly food, 78, 79
My HD Contract, 45, 56, 59, 238–39

Nori, 17, 80, 81
 Nori Vegetable Hummus Wrap, 227
 Nori Vegetable Wrap, 227
 Roasted Chia Nori Strips, 228
 Salmon Salad Nori Wrap, 214
 Seaweed Popcorn, 229
Nut allergies, 132, 135
Nutmeg
 Nutmeg Pumpkin Mash with Walnuts, 223
Nuts. *See also* Almond butter; Almond milk; Chia nut butter; Peanut butter
 as block food, 14
 choosing, 248
 Nutmeg Pumpkin Mash with Walnuts, 223

Oats and oatmeal
 Apple-Cinnamon Oatmeal, 172
 as block food, 12, 142
 Chia-Oat Pancake, 177
 gluten sensitivity and, 134
 as hydrophilic food, 12
 Quick Cacao Chia Oatmeal, 173
 Quick Chia Oatmeal, 173
 types of, 12–13
 While-You-Sleep Chia Oatmeal, 174
Obesity, 5, 120
Okra, 12
 HD Ratatouille, 200
 Lima Bean-Okra Soup, 197
Olive oil, calories in, 88
Omega-3 fatty acids, 11, 78–79, 119
Onion powder
 Onion Yogurt Dip, 182
On-the-Go Gobbler diet character, 32–33, 44, 47, 47–48, 57
Oranges, as hydrophilic food, 16
Oregano
 Lemon-Oregano Dressing, 190
Overeating, reasons for, 30, 31

Pancake
 Chia-Oat Pancake, 177
Parenting, as excuse for self-neglect, 150
Parsnips
 Parsnip Fries, 202
Pasta, white, as infrequent food, 124–25
Peanut butter
 Jicama-Nut Sandwich, 225
 Peanut Butter Cup Agar Pudding, 220
Pears, 13
 Poached Cinnamon Pears, 232
Pectin, 8, 13, 16
Pizza, as infrequent food, 125
Plump Know-It-All diet character, 35–36, 51, 51–52
Polyunsaturated fat, 78–79
Popcorn
 Different Ways to Make HD Popcorn, 229
Portion control, "Cheat Sheet" plate for, 89–90, **90**, 92, 107, 119, 171
Poultry. *See* Chicken; Turkey
Precontemplation, in Stages of Change model, 23–24
Preparation, in Stages of Change model, 24
Probiotics, for digestive health, 138
Processed foods
 ill effects of, 5, 138
 as infrequent foods, 118–19, 134
 sodium in, 122, 122
Processed meats, as infrequent food, 119–20
Protein bars, shakes, and drinks, as health derailer, 39
Proteins
 beans as, 15
 counting, 95
 HD-friendly, 76, 134
 high-hydrophilic, 75–76, 134, 136, 159–60
 overeating, 34, 35, 143, 168
Puddings
 agar-based, 17
 Agar Pudding, 220
 Good Decisions Cacao Chia Pudding, 221
 Good Decisions Vanilla Chia Pudding, 221
Pumpkin
 Nutmeg Pumpkin Mash with Walnuts, 223

Quercetin, health benefits of, 13

Ramekins, 100
Raspberries
 Berry Swirl Yogurt, 219
 Chia-Raspberry Smash, 185
 Free Frozen Fruit Skewer, 222
 Raspberry-Cacao Sorbet, 233
Ratatouille
 HD Ratatouille, 200

Recipes, 171. *See also specific recipes*
Red meat, as infrequent food, 119
Refined sweets, as infrequent foods, 120–21
Refined white flour, ill effects of, 5, 124
Restaurant meals, 37–38, 90, 127, 143, 152
Roasting vegetables, 167
Rosemary
  Rosemary-Lemon Salmon, 213

S

Saboteurs, of HD living, 148
Salad dressings, Good Decisions, 71, 189
  Balsamic Mustard Dressing, 189
  Lemon-Oregano Dressing, 190
  Miso Dressing, 191
  Salsa Dressing, 192
Salads
  Arame and Kale Salad, 186
  Asparagus and Artichoke Salad, 187
  beans as protein in, 15
  Broccoli-Red Cabbage Slaw, 188
  HD Tuna Salad, 215
  mistakes in making, 161
  Ultimate HD Salad, 92, 161–64
Salmon
  Chia-Crusted Salmon, 212
  Rosemary-Lemon Salmon, 213
  Salmon Salad Nori Wrap, 214
Salsa
  Salsa Dressing, 192
Salt
  cutting back on, 122
  as infrequent food, 121–23
  in recipes, 171
Satiety, 6, 8, 11, 74, 76, 77. *See also* HD satiation
Saturated fat, 114, 115, 119, 136
Sautéing vegetables, 166–67
Scallops
  Scallop Stir-Fry Shirataki, 217
Seaweeds, 80–81, 138
Seeds, choosing, 248
Self-control, for avoiding temptations, 153
Setbacks, excusitis and, 146
Sex life, exercise improving, 140–41
Shirataki noodles, 81, 245
  Scallop Stir-Fry Shirataki, 217
Side dishes
  HD Ratatouille, 200
  Mashed Turnips, 201
  Parsnip Fries, 202
  Spaghetti Squash, 203
  Sweet Potato Fries, 204
  Sweet Potato Roast, 204
  Zucchini "Fettuccine," 205
Slaw
  Broccoli-Red Cabbage Slaw, 188
Smoothie
  Chia Smoothie, 224
Snack foods, as infrequent foods, 123–24
Snacks
  Agar Pudding, 220
  Avocado Eggs, 230
  Chia Smoothie, 224
  Different Ways to Make HD Popcorn, 229
  failing to prepare, 37, 39
  Free Frozen Fruit Skewer, 222
  Good Decisions Cacao Chia Pudding, 221
  Good Decisions Vanilla Chia Pudding, 221
  guilt-free, 42, 102, 106
  in HD eating plan, 65
  Jicama-Nut Sandwich, 225
  Kale Chips, 226
  Nori Vegetable Wrap, 227
  Nutmeg Pumpkin Mash with Walnuts, 223
  Poached Cinnamon Pears, 232
  Raspberry-Cacao Sorbet, 233
  Roasted Chia Nori Strips, 228
  Roasted Chickpeas, 231
  Yogurts the HD Way, 219
Soapwort, uses for, 9
Soaring in HD phase, of HD eating plan, 69–70
Social life, as excuse for unhealthy eating, 152
Sodium, 120, 121–23
Sorbet
  Raspberry-Cacao Sorbet, 233
Soups
  Broccoli Soup, 193
  Gazpacho Soup, 194
  Good Decisions Soup, 195
  Lentil Soup, 196
  Lima Bean-Okra Soup, 197
  reduced-sodium broths, 84
  Vegetable-Chia Miso Soup, 198
Spaghetti squash
  Spaghetti Squash, 203
Special occasions, HD principles for handling, 147
Special requests, for restaurant meals, 143, 152
Spices, 82
Spinach
  Spinach Turkey Burgers, 218
  steamed vs. sautéed, 88
Squash
  Bean-Stuffed Acorn Squash, 206
  Spaghetti Squash, 203
  types of, 71
Stages of Change model, for new habit formation, **23**, 23–24
Start Strong phase, of HD eating plan, 66–67, 73, 85, 135
  easing into, 91
  eliminating red meat in, 119
  14-day menu plan for, 91–92, 92–99
  sample food log for, 55, 55
Steamer basket, 100
Steaming foods, 100, 166

Stevia, 82, 121, 142
Still Focused in HD phase, of HD eating plan, 68–69, 110–11, 125
Stir-fry
  Scallop Stir-Fry Shirataki, 217
Success stories. *See* HD success stories
Sugar, dependence on, 120–21
Supermarket, navigating, 243–48
Supplements, 137–38, 155
Sweet cravings, 17, 113, 121
Sweeteners
  artificial, 35, 82, 113–14, 142
  natural, 121
Sweet potatoes
  Sweet Potato Fries, 204
  Sweet Potato Roast, 204
Sweets
  guilt-free treats, 106
  refined, as infrequent food, 120–21
Swiss chard
  Swiss Chard Mini Frittatas, 180

Takeout foods, overreliance on, 33
Teas, 84
3-day diet recall, 27–28, 29, 30–32, 40
Tofu, 136
  Baked Tofu, 216
  Tofu Scrambler, 181
Tomatoes
  Gazpacho Soup, 194
Trans fats, 114–15
Triphala, for colon cleaning, 138
Truvia. *See* Stevia
Tuna
  HD Tuna Salad, 215
Turkey
  choosing, 248
  Spinach Turkey Burgers, 218
  Turkey Chili, 199
Turnips
  Mashed Turnips, 201

Vanilla extract
  Good Decisions Vanilla Chia Pudding, 221
  Vanilla Agar Pudding, 220
Vegans, 136
Vegetables. *See also specific vegetables*
  blanching, 166
  choosing, 243–44, 245–46
  cruciferous, cancer protection from, 15
  crudité, 165
  Good Decisions Soup, 195
  HD-friendly, 72
  high-hydrophilic, 70–71
  as freebie foods, 106
  gluten-free, 70–71, 134
  for salads, 161–62, 163–64
  steaming, 100
  for wraps, 165
  Nori Vegetable Hummus Wrap, 227
  Nori Vegetable Wrap, 227
  preparation methods for, 101, 166–67
  storing, 101
  Vegetable-Chia Miso Soup, 198
Vegetarians, 136

Wakame, 80, 81
Walnuts
  Nutmeg Pumpkin Mash with Walnuts, 223
Water, 83, 84, 112
Water retention, from salt, 122
Weekly goals, 59–60
Weekly Goal Tracker, 59, 242
Weigh-ins, 56, 58–59
Weight loss
  agar for, 17
  analogies about, 21–23
  changing habits for, 238
  daily decisions for, 23
  difficulty with, 6
  digestive health improving, 8
  insoluble fiber unsuitable for, 7
  realistic expectations for, 60
  stages for achieving, 23–25, 23
Weight management, 6, 139–40
Weight-tracking reports, 56, 58–59
  sample, of diet characters, 57, 58, 59
Wine, controlling consumption of, 148–49
Wraps
  building, 164–65
  Nori Vegetable Hummus Wrap, 227
  Nori Vegetable Wrap, 227
  Salmon Salad Nori Wrap, 214
Writing about goals and food decisions, 43–45

Yogurt
  dairy-free, 135
  Greek, 78, 135
  Yogurt Dip, 182
  Yogurts the HD Way, 219

Zucchini
  Nori Vegetable Wrap, 227
  Zucchini "Fettuccine," 205